MAKING IT THROUGH
THE STORM

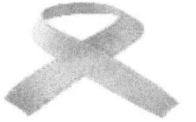

By TAMARA B. NEWBORN

Contents

DEDICATION 1

THANK YOU 2

I CAN! 5

    SIX MONTHS PRIOR TO MY STORM.. 6
    THE BEGINNING OF MY STORM 10

I WILL! 21

    CHAPTER 1 - FIRST CHEMO APPOINTMENT 22
    CHAPTER 2 - SECOND CHEMO APPOINTMENT - OCTOBER 6, 2017 42
    CHAPTER 3 - THIRD CHEMO TREATMENT - OCTOBER 20, 2017 48
    CHAPTER 4 - FOURTH CHEMO TREATMENT - NOVEMBER 3, 2017 55
    CHAPTER 5 - FIFTH CHEMO TREATMENT - NOVEMBER 17, 2017 64
    CHAPTER 6 - SIXTH CHEMO TREATMENT - DECEMBER 1, 2017 70
    CHAPTER 7 - SEVENTH CHEMO TREATMENT - DECEMBER 15, 2017 78
    CHAPTER 8 - EIGHTH AND FINAL TREATMENT - JANUARY 5, 2018 85

I MUST! 88

    CHAPTER 9 - DOUBLE MASTECTOMY - JANUARY 23, 2018 89
    CHAPTER 10 - POST OPERATION APPOINTMENT WITH MY BREAST
    SPECIALIST 92
    CHAPTER 11 - EXPANSION APPOINTMENTS 95
    CHAPTER 12 - RADIATION – MARCH 20, 2018 98
    CHAPTER 13 – XELODA/RADIATION RECALL... 106
    CHAPTER 14 - RECONSTRUCTIVE SURGERY 117

I DID! 122

    CHAPTER 15 – I MADE IT THROUGH THE STORM 124
    CHAPTER 16 – THINGS I LEARNED WHILE GOING THROUGH THE STORM .. 126
    CHAPTER 17 - GOING THROUGH THE STORM.. 133

Dedication

**Dedicated to my mother, Pearlie Mae Brand.
November 28, 2017**

    To the person that I ran to with every problem that I had no matter how big or small it was. To the person who knew me better than I knew myself. To my first teacher, the first person who I loved and who loved me back, and my soap opera buddy. Now here I am fighting the biggest battle of my life, and you are unable to make it easier because you are busy fighting a battle of your own.

    Mom you knew my potential, and because of it you always made me strive for more even when I didn't understand why. When I was in college pursuing my master's, I asked you why I was continuing when I wasn't even working in that career field, and you told me to continue so that when God sent my "calling," I would be ready. I never understood that until now. Throughout my fifty years of school, I acquired the ability and passion to put pen to paper, and now I am able to use that "calling" to tell my testimony. I love you mom, and I'll make you proud by fighting this battle while keeping the faith like you taught me to.

    Psalm 118:17 (KJV) - I shall not die, but live, and declare the works of the LORD.

Thank you

First and foremost, I thank the Lord above for giving me the strength to make it through my darkest days. Through God's grace, I was able to keep it moving when I didn't think it was possible. I am thankful to inspirational people like Pastor Joel Osteen who I listened to when I needed reassurance that what I was going through was all part of God's plan. I am thankful for Pastor John Gray for those days that I needed to hear the word, but I didn't want to be emotional while doing so. Being able to laugh while hearing the word was helpful. Lastly, I'd like to thank motivational speaker Dr. Eric Thomas for reminding me that I Can! I Will! I Must! When I was too tired to see that one day I'd be able to say I did! Listening to their words gave me the strength to fight hard enough so that I am able to stand here today shouting I kicked cancer's butt!!

I'd like to thank a friend that I met and lost during this battle. We met during chemo and motivated each other until God called her home. Her motivation and kind words kept me strong when I was weak. RIP J!!

Lastly, I would like to thank the best family in the world for making me feel normal when I didn't look it. Extra special thanks to my sisters: Tina Harper and Marsha Brand Hester, who were always there when I needed ya; My niece Miranda Hester who had my prayer wall swagged out with her handwritten poster boards of my mom's favorite scriptures and for texting me daily the week of chemo to check on me; 3 Dimension Studios Designs for my t-shirts with those scripture that I wore to every chemo appointment; my in-laws for being there for my appointments and surgeries; and, last but definitely not least, my children, Kylee and Kameron who never made me feel bad when I was too weak to do and my husband, Kelsey Newborn, who helped me kick cancer's butt like we were fighting nothing more than a common cold. I thank you for staying the course.

Special thank you to all of these organizations:

Sisters Network of Dallas

IGOPINK/Help Now Fund

Women Rock

Cleaning for a Reason

The Pink Fund

Catherine H. Tuck Foundation

Patient Advocate Foundation

Copay Relief Program

Baylor Scott and White

Texas Oncology

Reba Ranch House

Because of you, I was able to concentrate on getting better while going through the storm

Psalm 30:2 (KJV) – "O LORD my God, I cried unto thee, and thou hast healed me."

I CAN!

2 Timothy 1:7 (KJV) *- For God hath not given us the spirit of fear; but of power, and of love, and of a sound mind.*

Six Months Prior to My Storm

Sixth months prior to my storm, I was dealing with my mother's storm. Towards the end of 2016 and early part of 2017, my mother's health had begun declining. She was in bed most of the day, and when I talked to her on the phone, she would say things like "she wasn't feeling good" or "she was tired," but she always downplayed the severity of her situation. I can count the number of times on one hand that I saw my mother sick over the years, so I knew if she actually admitted not feeling good, then it wasn't good.

My mom had told me about a lump in her breast six months prior, so I worried that the lump was the cause of her discomfort. I knew that if the lump was causing her pain and discomfort there was a big possibility that it was cancerous. When she first told me about her lump, she told me that she wouldn't be getting any medical attention for it. Instead, she decided that she would pray to the Lord for healing. When the lump and the pain from it got worse, she decided to start a home remedy instead of seeking medical attention. Unfortunately, the remedy didn't help, and her health continued to decline.

My family begged her to seek medical attention which she rejected. Knowing that my mother was against medical care, I hated asking her to seek treatment, but I knew that she was in pain and I was hoping that the doctor would give her medication to treat her pain. She continued to reject our requests for her to seek medical care and she continued to pray over her situation; meanwhile, her health drastically declined.

Most of my siblings who lived out of state were unaware of how bad my mother's condition really was. Whenever I called my mother, she would pretend that she was ok. She would tell us whatever we needed to hear so that we didn't worry about her.

Her health had gotten so bad that she eventually stopped taking our calls. I later found out that the breathing issue she had which was due to a fluid build-up in her lungs made it hard for her to talk on the phone.

Initially, it was very important for us to respect our mother's wishes so when she said she didn't want to seek medical treatment, we didn't push it. It was so hard to sit back and know that my mother was suffering when all she had to do was seek medical attention. After hearing from a family member near my mother about how bad her condition had gotten, a few of my siblings and I flew home to take her to the hospital.

When we made it to my mother's house, we were greeted by some of our cousins and my mother's siblings who were in town to urge her to seek medical attention as well. My mother was really adamant about not seeking treatment, so she declined her siblings' requests.

I remember the feeling when I first walked into my mother's house. The energy was off which I knew meant that things were worse than I expected. Looking into the faces of my mother's brothers and seeing sadness also confirmed my suspicions that my mother was not ok. When I walked into my mother's bedroom, I was shocked to see all of the things that were there that shouldn't have been. I remember seeing a toilet and a breathing treatment machine that I had no idea that she was using. Seeing a toilet in her bedroom meant that my mother was confined to her bedroom and I was unaware of that. It hurt to know that my mother was struggling and I wasn't there when she needed me most.

After my siblings and I begged and pleaded with my mother to go to the hospital, she agreed to let the ambulance take her. We walked the halls of the hospital for hours that night waiting on feedback about my mother's health. We heard a lot of suspicions from different people but nothing concrete. I even overheard a doctor on the phone with someone saying that my mother had breast cancer and pneumonia. All we were told that night was that they were admitting her so that they could run more tests. They gave her pain meds to help her with the pain that was being caused by the lump that had begun protruded through her bruised breast.

The doctors eventually diagnosed my mother with metastatic cancer. By the time she made it to the hospital, the cancer that started in her breast had spread to other parts of her body. I remember sitting in her room thinking about how her late diagnosis could have contributed to her late-stage cancer. To possibly avoid that diagnosis myself, I knew that I needed to seek care.

The doctors requested that my mother take chemotherapy to prolong her life pass the 6 months that they gave her without it but she declined. She declined chemo and told us that she wanted to continue to lean on the Lord.

Hearing her say that she wouldn't take the chemo was hard. All I could think about was that she had a chance to prolong her life to be with us and she wasn't taking it. I failed to realize that this wasn't about me. My mom had raised her children and helped raise several others, and it was only right that she put herself first and she was doing so by solely leaning on God. It was hard to think about the consequences of her decision, but I accepted that it was her decision to make.

I have since learned that when it comes to cancer treatment there is no right answer. You can either go the traditional route by receiving treatment or the nontraditional route by not and leaning on the Lord. Accepting that she was declining chemo treatment meant that I had to accept that there was a big chance that she wouldn't make it to see the next year. I knew that I had to be ok with that, so I continuously prayed for strength to make it through those days when the time came.

For the next couple of months, we heard a lot of bad news from the doctors, so I was constantly reminding my mother that God has the last say. When the prognosis became harder for her to hear, I would remind her that the doctors talked about science and medicine, but we focused on the word of the higher power. This always helped her because even though she acted unaffected, it was obvious that all of the bad news was draining her emotionally.

The Beginning of my Storm

Over a year before I was diagnosed, while conducting a home breast exam looking for any "911" issues, I felt something very small poking against the inside of my right breast. Over the next year, I convinced myself that the small lump that I discovered was nothing. Family members who I told about the lump pressured me to go to the doctor. This was a stressful time because even though I knew I needed to go, I was scared. I was scared to hear that the lump that I had convinced myself was benign wasn't. I wasn't ready to hear those words. My husband was very concerned and asked me several times to go get it checked. Because he is not the type to pressure me to make decisions, I continued to talk myself out of doing what I knew was right by getting it checked. I let the fear set in and for a year, I watched the lump grow bigger. I had a grandma, aunt, and older sister who were all diagnosed with cancer but instead of that knowledge pushing me to go get myself checked, I let it scare me.

In the summer of 2016, I remember talking to my mother about the lump that I discovered in my right breast. I was shocked to find out from her that she had also discovered a lump in the same breast. She told me to pray over the lump because that was what she decided to do. She was a firm believer in speaking things into existence. She told me that I shouldn't be trying to claim any issues. So I didn't. I was already scared, so I took comfort in talking to her about it because she wasn't pressuring me into doing something that I knew that I needed to do but was too scared to. I'm not sure how long it had been since she had discovered her lump, but I got the impression that she discovered it long before I discovered mine. We discussed going to the doctor. I asked her why she was against getting her breast checked and she told me because God hadn't put it on her heart to do so. She went on to talk about a lump that she once had on her hand. She said she prayed over that lump and it went away. She told me to go get my lump checked if that's where the Lord was leading me but that she wouldn't be doing so. She said she was leaning on her faith and prayed that God would remove the lump. Hearing her talk about leaning on her faith instead of getting checked confused me. I knew that if I was ever diagnosed with cancer that I would be receiving treatment, but I didn't want that to mean that I didn't believe in God's will. I began dealing with another dilemma. Which was - Should I go and get the results of my lump or should I take the route that my mom was taking and continue to pray over it in hopes that it would go away? I decided to pray. If my mom was doing it and she was ok, I thought, "I would be too."

It was almost seven months from my mother's diagnosis before I met with a doctor to seek medical care for myself. I helped in caring for my mother, so my attention was in taking care of her. Plus, I didn't think I really had reason to worry. Another lesson that I learned is, when in doubt check it out. I wish I would have checked it out sooner but I let the fear delay me and that lead to me having stage 2B breast cancer instead of 1 like my sister.

OBGYN Appointment

Around August 28, 2017, I scheduled an OBGYN appointment to have my annual visit and fo finally have the tumor checked. When I first discovered the tumor, it was really small but by the time I laid on the table of my OBGYN's office, it had more than tripled in size.

I picked my children up from school that day and headed to the doctor. I originally planned to pick them up from school and drop them off at home on the way to my appointment just in case I got bad news and was emotional on the way home. Unfortunately, I left work late so I ran late to pick them up. They sat in the waiting room while I sat in the back waiting on the nurse practitioner. While all of this is going on, I'm worried about my mom who was checked into the hospital a couple of hours earlier for breathing complications, severe headaches, and blurry vision. I was also worried that my tumor could actually be cancer instead of a benign tumor.

I prayed to God that my family wouldn't be hit this hard twice in one year. After waiting 20 minutes and scaring myself half to death worrying about my mother's condition and the possibility of having cancer myself, I decided I had to get out of there. As long as I didn't get a diagnosis, I wouldn't have to worry about what came next, and I would be able to give all my attention to helping care for my mom. I got up off the bed and stuck my head outside the door to where the nurses' station was, and I told the nurse sitting there that I needed to get to my mom. I told them that I had no problems rescheduling that I just wanted to get where she was. I knew that there was nothing that I could do for her but being close would help me stay calm. I was told that the nurse practitioner would be in any minute. To be honest, I was hoping that they would give me the out that I so desperately needed to reschedule my appointment. It had been over a year since I discovered the lump and I still wasn't ready to have it diagnosed. I was looking for any reason possible to prolong the inevitable. I was so freaking scared and so freaking worried, so I'd say and do anything to reschedule. When the nurse practitioner came in, she asked about my mom being in the hospital and was obviously shocked to hear that she was in the hospital suffering from the disease that I was there to see if I had. We talked for a few minutes longer about my family's history with cancer. I told her that my paternal grandma, aunt, and sister had all been previously diagnosed with cancer. She then asked me to change into one of those ugly hospital gowns, and after performing an uncomfortable pap smear, she started her examination of the breast where I had the lump. We discussed how long I had the lump, any pains from it that I may or may not have, and if it had grown in size since I first noticed it. She was aware of how scared I was. On top of me letting her know several times that I was scared, I'm sure she knew that my mother, sister, and grandma's diagnosis with breast cancer in the same breast didn't help.

Even though she tried to hide it, I knew the moment she realized that my tumor might be a problem. When her tone of voice changed, I asked if she felt the tumor and what she thought. She told me that she felt the lump, but she said that she wasn't sure that it was something for me to be concerned about. She said that because of my family's history it was best for me to get it looked at. She gave me a list of places to choose from to have the mammogram and ultrasound done. I don't know why but hearing her say that she didn't think that the lump was anything to be concerned about was comforting even though I knew that it wouldn't be that easy. She told me how important it was to get the mammogram and the ultrasound done as soon as possible because the breast specialist that she wanted me to see couldn't see me until I had them both done.

After the appointment, I called my sister to check on my mother. I was told that she was ok but that she was checked into the hospital where they would be conducting more tests. Not getting the peace from my appointment and hearing that my mother was checked into the hospital left me emotionally drained. On top of stressing about scheduling my mammogram, I was worried about my mom and her tests.

We were eventually told that the headaches and blurry visions that my mom had been experiencing were caused by cancerous lesions that were now in her brain. Her oncologist continuously urged her to take chemo which she was still opposed to, but she agreed to begin a radiation treatment on her brain. We were told that this would help the cancerous lesions. Throughout everything that my mother was enduring, she still refused to admit that she had cancer.

Now that being diagnosed with cancer was becoming more real I wanted to talk to my mother about it, but I knew that I couldn't. I knew that there was no way that I could talk to her about my concerns when she was still in denial of her diagnosis, so I didn't. This was the biggest personal storm that I had ever faced, and for once I was unable to talk to the person who always made me feel better. My mother would always tell me not to worry about whatever storm I was facing while praying and given me the peace that I needed and I so needed that from her.

Mammogram and Ultrasound Appointment

After weeks of worrying about my lump and putting off scheduling my appointment with the radiologists, I finally made it to the appointment where I had the mammogram and the ultrasound of my lump done. I knew I needed to be prepared because it was a possibility that after this appointment my life would be changed forever.

I sat in the waiting room sipping a cup of coffee that I had just poured pretending that this appointment would be like any other appointment when I heard my name being called.

The nurse and I talked about basic things on the way down the long hallway that would lead us to the dressing room. When we got there, the nurse asked me to change into a gown and come into the room where the mammogram would be performed. When I was dressed, I walked into the cold, gloomy, room with the big machine and started the mammogram procedure. The nurse and I both talked about our daughters who were in the fifth grade. In the school district that we were in, fifth graders attended a camp for 3 days. She talked about her daughter attending the camp in a week or so while I was hoping that my daughter wouldn't have to go for a while. I didn't know how my health would be at the time, and because of that, I worried. I could tell she probably felt bad for me and my situation. "Here I was with a daughter who would possibly be attending camp following her mother's passing." At one point while taking the pictures, she stopped and left the room. She told me that she needed to go ask the radiologists a question. I knew that wasn't normal so I was sure that she saw something that she knew she needed to discuss with the doctor. After the mammogram, we did the ultrasound. She tried to sound normal but like before; I could tell when she noticed something that could be a problem. She stopped performing the ultrasound and left the room. She came back with the doctor who watched her go over the spots in my breast that may be a problem. Because they both were so quiet, I knew there was a problem. I asked if everything was ok and I was told by the doctor that I need to hurry and schedule an appointment with the breast specialist because the tumors that were shown on the screen was troubling. At that moment, it went from one to two. She also told me that there was another issue that I hadn't realized. It was the spot near my arms. Hearing that I possibly had so many tumors and because of it my situation may be a lot worse, instantly made me emotional. I was hoping that what the nurse told me a couple of weeks back was true and that I didn't have anything to worry about, but I was being told by the radiologists that I definitely had something to worry about and that it was urgent for me to seek treatment. Tears began streaming down my face as I half listened to what the radiologist was saying. Seeing the look of sadness on both of their faces only made things worse. Everything after that moment was a blur. I remember them asking me if I was ok and me telling them no but I would be.

At that moment I was so weak. I didn't know how I'd find the strength to be ok, but I knew that I would be. When I got outside, I called my husband who didn't answer, so I immediately called my sister who I knew was sitting with my mother for the day. Through blurred vision, I was able to dial her number. After making sure that she wasn't in the room with my mother, I told her that the doctor had just told me that I had cancer! My sister was diagnosed and beat cancer 5 years prior, so she knew that a diagnosis was not a death sentence but like me, she wasn't ready to hear those words. She instantly prayed for me on the phone. The harder she prayed, the more I cried. She told me that she was on the way before hanging up.

Before leaving work the day before, I told my supervisor that I had a doctor's appointment and that I would be in after so I knew I needed to call and update her. When I called to tell her that I wouldn't be in for the day, I began crying. All I could think about was what I had just been told by the radiologist. I told her what I was told and of course she was speechless. I knew I needed to take the day to deal with what I'd been told before having to tell my children.

My sister showed up at my house along with two other sisters and my youngest brother. We sat on my couch for several hours just talking and in shock. They were doing what I needed them to do by telling me that I could and would beat this. I knew that I had the strength to do so, but I just didn't want to have to fight. I talked to them about worrying about getting sick while going through chemo, about losing my hair and scaring my children. At that time, those were all big concerns of mine. We went from talking about my mom and her situation to my sister and her victory. While they tried pretending otherwise, I knew that they were all as petrified as I was. We all knew that God was in control, but the unknown is always a scary thing.

My sister came to visit me the following morning on her way back home to Mississippi because she wanted to "lay her eyes on me" before she headed out. My family is big on "laying our eyes" on each other. When one of us goes through a storm and tells the other that we are ok, we are not comfortable until we look that person in the eyes to gauge for ourselves.

We sat on the couch talking about the journey that I was getting ready to take. See my sister had been diagnosed and beat breast cancer over 5 years before, so she knew what it took. I told her that I wasn't ready and she told me that I had no choice but to get ready. She told me that she knew that I was strong enough to make it through. I told her that I knew that I had the strength and that I would fight with the best of my ability but that I didn't want to have to fight. My sister was in a similar situation as me when she was diagnosed. She had a young son and daughter that she had to fight to make it for. We both had too much to live for to not give this fight our all.

Diagnosed with Breast Cancer

While most doctors don't recommend that their patients have a mammogram until the age of 40, at 36 I was diagnosed with breast cancer. I knew that being diagnosed with breast cancer was not a death sentence, but it was definitely something that I didn't want to hear. I remember sitting on the table in my doctor's office with tears streaming down my face. While she was discussing possible treatment options, I was stuck thinking, "It's real!" What I thought wouldn't happen to me was happening. I could no longer feel comfortable with the lie that I had been telling myself over the last year about the tumor that I found in my right breast. I now knew that the tumor that I convinced myself was benign wasn't, which meant that I actually had breast cancer!

I looked over to my husband who was sitting in the nearest chair with a dazed look on his face. While the doctor was telling me things that I needed to know about my diagnosis, I had zoned out so I heard none of it. Instead, I thought back to what my radiologist had told me the day before.

> **Reflecting back to my Radiology Appointment -**
> "The tumors that I see on the screen are very troubling. I see the one that you are concerned with, but I also see tumors near your lymph nodes." Until that moment, I didn't think that I had to worry about

my lymph nodes. When my sister was diagnosed with breast cancer, she was told that the cancer had spread to her lymph nodes so I knew that wasn't good. The radiologists went on to talk to me about the urgency of seeing my breast doctor. Because of that appointment, I knew that it was highly likely that I had breast cancer, but I still wasn't prepared to hear it from my doctor.

I stared at my doctor with the same dazed look that my husband held. Tears were streaming down my face. "What was I going to do?" I thought. I understood what she was telling me, but I still wanted to live in denial. I knew that she was sure about my diagnosis, but I wanted to keep hope alive until I received the results of my biopsy that she had yet to perform. My doctor not wanting to destroy my little bit of hope, sadly looked at me and said, "I've been doing this for years, so I know that this is breast cancer but I will call you tomorrow when I get the results, and I'll give you your treatment plan then." I'm sure she was trying to give me hope when she knew that there was no reason to. I began thinking like my mom who was diagnosed a few months earlier, "I can't claim this!" I repeated this over and over to myself.

After discussing my family's history with cancer, my doctor asked me to take the BRCA genetic test which would let me know if my cancer was hereditary. I repeatedly told her "no" that I wouldn't be doing it. I was both scared and overwhelmed. She wanted me to make decisions that I was just not in a great headspace to make. After calming me down and addressing all of my concerns, my doctor stepped out for a minute to give my husband and me time to grasp what we were just told.

I remember both of us staring at each other looking dumbfounded. We were so clueless. We were unsure of what to say, how to feel, or what to do. We were just told news that would break the strongest person. We both knew that we needed to be strong but "how!" we wondered. I remember jumping from the bed that I was sitting on while talking to my doctor and running to my phone so that I could text my family through our group chat to let them know everything that my doctor had just told me. Even though I knew there was nothing that they could do, I needed to let them know that my worry was now a reality. I think I also needed to hear them say it was ok and that I was strong enough to fight this battle because I was panicking. My breathing was short, and my adrenaline was amplified. "What would happen now?" is all I could think. My husband, who knows me so well, knew that I was panicking. He grabbed my hands and with tears in his eyes told me that we were going to get through this. This calmed me enough to do what we knew was customary when going through a storm; we prayed. We prayed for God to give us the strength to make it through this storm just as we had every storm prior.

Dreaded Biopsy procedure

When my doctor came back in the room, she sent my husband to the waiting room while she prepared to perform what would become my most emotional procedure, the biopsy. I think this procedure was so emotional because it was the moment that I subconsciously accepted that the life that I dreaded for over a year was now my reality. I was a 36-year-old wife, mother, sister, and daughter, diagnosed with breast cancer and my life as I knew it would never be the same. This meant that on top of chemo treatments, I would have to have a couple of major surgeries. I've often heard of women having to have a biopsy, but I never imagined that I would be one of those women and definitely not at the age of 36.

This experience is different for every woman. I've heard women say that it wasn't painful at all, but for me, it was very painful. I remember squirming and whining on the table while my doctor performed the procedure. It seemed the deeper she delved into my skin, the more it hurt. I had no idea where she was inside of me or why but I can say that it was extremely uncomfortable. Yes, I was given numbing meds, and because of it, I was told that I shouldn't feel any pain, but I did. I was unable to see exactly what she was doing because I was laid back with my hands behind my head while she sat next to me conducting the biopsy. From the pain that was being caused and how steady she worked, I imagined that she was carving the inside of my breast like you would carve a pumpkin for Halloween. Dramatic, yes I know, but that's how I felt. At one part during the procedure, I remember sighing and telling my doctor that it was painful and being told by her that it was all in my head because the medication should have me too numb to feel anything. Regardless of what pain meds that I was given, I knew that I was in pain, but I also knew that I had to finish this procedure so I continued to lay there hoping that she would be done soon. After reaching out to her several times to stop her from the pain she was causing, I was treated like a child, and my arm was held still by one of the nurses. The doctor explained my tumor markers, but my head was everywhere but there listening to her, so I'm still not sure what she said.

I knew that I had to let go and let God so again I laid back and closed my eyes and pondered how much my life had changed over the last year. Instead of still being in law school and worrying about test scores, I was now at my doctor's office and I was worried about my health scores. Now, Instead of worrying about passing quizzes, tests, and the bar to become an attorney, I was worried about passing chemo, surviving my double mastectomy, and radiation to become a survivor. I began quoting all of the scriptures that I heard my mom recite over the years. I needed strength and I knew that God was the only one that could give it to me.

I WILL!

Isaiah 41:10 *- "Fear thou not; for I am with thee: be not dismayed; for I am thy God: I will strengthen thee; yea, I will help thee; yea, I will uphold thee with the right hand of my righteousness."*

Chapter 1 - First Chemo Appointment

Feeling Overwhelmed

The call from my doctor confirming my results is when it all started. I had my biopsy performed the day before. My doctor told me that she knew I had cancer but that she would call me after she received the results from the lab. It was almost 4 pm the following day when I heard from her.

I was at work and beginning to relax when I looked down and saw her number incoming on my cellphone. She told me that she had my results and asked if it was a good time to discuss them. I knew that I was getting ready to hear news from her that I didn't want to hear so there was no reason to put it off. I stepped into my boss's office and talked to her. She explained my results and how it confirmed her suspicions that I had breast cancer. She continued talking about the results, but I blocked out everything she said because once again I was stuck at the part where she said that I had breast cancer. I started to tear up while asking her if she thought I could beat it. She told me that as long as I followed the treatment plan that she was about to give me that I would be fine. That's when she discussed who my oncologist would be. She told me that my oncologist would take his own scans and work up a treatment plan. Before hanging up, she assured me that someone from his office would be calling me the following morning. I remember going back to my cubicle and gathering my things to leave for the day. I had a lot to process before picking my kids up for the day. I was emotional, and I couldn't let them see me in that state. I knew that I was getting ready to fight one of the hardest battles of my life to make sure they weren't motherless children. I knew that our initial conversation about this would set the tone for our journey and I didn't want it to be full of me crying. I imagined that would only scare them and send them into panic mode. It was hard for me to hear those same words about my mother but at least I was grown when I had to hear them. My mother and I had a very close relationship, so it was hard for me to fathom losing her. For days on end, I continuously prayed for her health and healing. When her health worsened, I prayed harder. When I had doctors telling me that there was no way that she would get better, I prayed harder. I prayed harder than I had ever prayed before but several months later, not only was I having to accept the reality that I was losing my mother, I was also having to accept that I was being diagnosed with breast cancer too. The worst part is when I was diagnosed I felt all prayed out, so I had little prayer left for myself.

The Fight

"How much can one person handle?" I remember thinking while crying a river full of tears the night that I was told by my doctor that I had cancer. I was already failing at dealing with my mother's diagnosis. I tortured myself by spending that night laying in the dark looking at videos of people who were diagnosed and their journey. In order to make it through it, I had to know what I would be facing. Yes, my sister fought and won her battle over 5 years prior and my mother was battling the disease at the same time, but neither of their journeys put my mind at ease. My sister lived over 6 hours away, so I wasn't close enough to watch her go through the fight and win her battle. I remember her being very emotional days after each chemo treatment, but I didn't know much about what the appointments entailed. I also remember seeing her with no hair for the first time and how it felt to see her that way. I love my sister and seeing her with no hair scared me. I don't know if it made me feel like she'd lose her battle or not, but I know I didn't like it. One thing that I took away from my sister that day was her strength while going through her storm. She smiled when others would have cried. She embodied a strength that I never knew she had. I knew I had to dig deep within myself and embrace that same strength and confidence if I was going to make it through my storm. I knew that my family would look at me the same way so I had to be strong in order for them to do so. With everything going on with my mother, I didn't want them to have to suffer seeing two people wither away.

While in the hospital immediately following her diagnosis, my mother endured two chemo treatments and because of it, she lost some of her hair, but it wasn't as drastic as the change that my sister endured. My mother lost a lot of weight after being diagnosed but I think the weight loss was due to the cancer eating away within her and nothing to do with the chemo treatments. My mother, for the most part, denied treatment, so I was unable to see the effects of treatment.

While watching my sister go through chemo and surgery helped me to see how a strong person could successfully make it through the storm, it didn't put my mind at ease about what to expect. Looking at the videos both scared me and helped to put my mind at ease. I saw videos of ladies before and after their treatment. I saw women receiving their chemo treatments, radiation treatments, losing their hair, getting their chemo curls, and some of the women who were living years later cancer free. There is a celebrity who documented her journey with breast cancer. She had well-documented videos that showed her losing her hair all the way through to getting her chemo curls. While there were moments where the chemo had her down, there were also moments where she was happy and upbeat. Seeing her videos was scary but helpful and informative because they were so raw. Her videos showed her as a cancer patient and not as the celebrity I was used to seeing. I remember watching one of her videos after she had endured a couple of rounds of chemotherapy and she had begun losing her hair. Even though losing her hair was a big blow she was still strong and full of fight. We saw her get her hair cut short before the chemo was in her system and she began losing it in clumps. She talked about letting her mom cut her bald so emotionally she wouldn't have to worry about waking up daily to clumps of hair on her pillow. She was able to smile while going through the storm and I prayed that I'd be able to do the same. By the end of that night, I had made a decision to fight this battle head-on. I would go through this journey with a will to fight. I knew that it wouldn't be an easy battle, but I knew that no matter how hard it got I wouldn't crumple without giving it the fight of my life. I thought, "I made it through so many storms in my life, and I intended to make it through this too."

From those videos and watching my sister fight her battle, I learned that for the most part, my personality would dictate my destiny. If I was sad and overwhelmed, my journey would be as such. I hoped if I was as upbeat as possible, I would be able to make it through this storm in the least amount of pain as possible. One thing that I learned from my sister when she was going through her battle was that my family would take their lead about how to feel and react from me. If I walked around sad and defeated, they would feel the same way when it came to my battle.

When my sister went through her battle, she was, for the most part, upbeat. Since she was upbeat, we stayed upbeat and didn't worry as much. I wanted to do that for my family who were already worried and stressing over my mother.

Even though I was the one diagnosed, I was worried about my family. I was sad for them. I hated it for my siblings and father who were already dealing with watching my mother deteriorate from the disease that was now living within me. I was sad for my husband and children because they were being thrown into a lifestyle that they didn't ask for. We had already lost a grandma, aunt, and several other family members to this disease. I was unsure how sick I was and because I was watching my mother I was imagining the worse. I imagined my husband having to take care of an ailing spouse and two innocent children standing by watching. I was sad for my children because I was unsure of the changes that lie ahead for them. I knew there was a possibility that they would have to live their lives without a mother at the age of 6 and 10. I thought about showing up at their soccer games and school events with a bald head and how embarrassing this would be for them. They were just young innocent kids, and I didn't want them to have to deal with those types of things. I prayed to God to shield them from the hard days. Being a mother meant that I had to protect my babies and now I was being thrown into a situation where I could possibly cause them pain. Going through this stage was so rough. My mind was being bombarded with superficial things such as: losing my hair and possibly losing a gain of weight.

I remember telling my co-workers that my biggest issue with being diagnosed was my children. I felt that they were getting ready to go through a storm and hard times that they didn't ask for and the hardest part was that I couldn't shield them from. Because of my diagnosis, they would be robbed of their innocence. They would be forced into a role that they weren't ready for. I failed to remember that there is always a purpose in our pain and that the lesson that was about to be taught was not only for me but was for my children as well. I didn't know what their lesson would be, but I prayed that whatever it was would put them on a path to becoming a stronger person. That it could also be used to help the next person going through this storm.

I knew that the storm that I was getting ready to go through wouldn't be easy, but I had no choice but to put my big girl panties on to make it through.

The weeks following my diagnosis consisted of the loneliest times of my life. Yes, I had my husband and other family members that I could talk to, but I didn't want to put that burden on them. I had so many doubts and worries in my mind but I knew leaning on my family would weaken and overload them, and I couldn't afford their worry in order to be strong. Plus, I didn't want them worrying about me because we all were working fulltime on caring for my mother. My siblings were worried and stressed about my mom's condition so I couldn't burden them.

I couldn't lean on my husband with my worries because I needed him to believe that I was strong in order for him to stay strong. At the time, that's what I thought I needed in order to make it through. I remember talking to my husband before starting chemo and telling him that I knew that I was getting ready to go through some hard days and I needed him to stay strong in order for me to make it through those days. I knew that as long as he didn't make it seem like we were going through a crisis situation, then I wouldn't feel like I was going through one. I asked him to fake being strong for me even if he wasn't. I hated asking that of him because while I may have been the one being diagnosed, he was also affected by the illness. He was dealing with our new reality, and the last thing that I wanted to do was overload him before he had a chance to get used to the change.

For the first time ever in my life, I felt alone. I later realized that God put me in that situation so that I learned to lean on him solely because He is who I would need to make it through the storm.

In the Beginning

The first couple of weeks after being diagnosed with breast cancer I was extremely emotional. All I wanted to do was cry, but I knew I couldn't. My mission was to win this battle, and I felt I could only do so by staying emotionally and mentally strong. My faith played a big part in helping me stay strong. I knew that I had to deal with every obstacle that I would endure as just that, an obstacle blocking me from my biggest blessing of healing. In the beginning, it was hard for me to say the word cancer, but I didn't have long to get used to it. I felt like I was diagnosed with breast cancer one day and the following 5 or so days I was called daily to schedule doctor appointments. I was told by my doctor that since I discovered my tumor so long before seeking help, it was possible that the cancer had spread outside of my breast and lymph nodes. The tests were needed to rule that out. I was still having a hard time dealing with my mother's metastatic battle with breast cancer and then being told that not only did I have cancer but the possibility of the cancer being metastasized was so stressful and scary.

I was scheduled for an MRI, CT scan, and an appointment with my new oncologist by the end of the first week. There were times where I didn't want to answer my phone because it was too overwhelming and all of these appointments pushed me to accept my new reality. I took every scan imaginable and thanked God they all came back negative besides the spots that I was already aware of. Because of the number of cases of cancer in my family, I was told that I needed to take genetic testing which I was originally against. I was also originally against a double mastectomy. In the beginning, I was against everything that was different than what I was used to. Family support helped a lot.

Family Support

I remember my older sister scheduling her MRI the same time that I did to support me. She knew that I was afraid of doctors and with everything that was going on with my mother she knew my mind was running and in the wrong direction. Her appointment was scheduled right before mine so by the time that I got there she was already back. I remember the secretary telling me that my sister told her that I would be coming in and to tell me that she was ok. See my sister knows how much of a worrier

I am. She also knows that I can be emotional and sensitive at times. By the time I got to the back and changed into the gown for my MRI she walked in. She told me that she was going in when I took my MRI. I knew that was against the rules so I knew that there was no way that she would be doing so. Little did I know, she had already told the person performing the MRI that I was recently diagnosed and about my mother's illness. My sister is very persuasive, and she used those skills to talk him into letting her come into the room as long as she sat in the corner which she was happy to do.

He started off telling me about having to put an IV in so that he could run a dye that would need to run through my body at some point through the MRI. I instantly panicked. I've always been afraid of needles, and now I was being told that I would have to endure the IV. This was before I knew how much poking and IV's I'd have to endure during this journey. After acting like a baby, I was able to sit still long enough to let him put the IV in my arm. That process was worse than the procedure. I went through the MRI without a problem. I vaguely remember him running the dye through my body. I just know that it was done because he let me know prior to doing it. I am so thankful to my sister for being there for me when I needed her. When I was younger, I hated being part of a big family. Now I was thanking God because I was getting ready to fight one of the biggest battles of my life and I needed their support to make it through.

I really thank my sister for coming to this visit because it was because of this visit, she later found out that she had breast cancer as well. This was when I realized that the storm that I was going through was not only for me but for my family too.

First Oncology Appointment - September 13, 2017

Once I finished all of my scans, my oncologist informed me of his recommended treatment plan. He wanted me to go through

4 rounds of chemo treatment then he would reassess to see how many more rounds I needed to endure. Both he and my breast specialists agreed that because of the large size of my tumor (5") that it was best for him to try to shrink the tumor before performing my surgery. This concerned me because my sister who was a breast cancer survivor and a couple of other family members of mine had a different treatment plan. They had their surgery then chemotherapy. In my head, a different plan meant different results and I wanted the results that my sister had. I wanted to one day be cancer free for five years and counting.

My oncologist went on to explain my pathology report and a couple of other things that would take place in the future, but he said we would worry about those things as time progressed which was a good thing because I was already overwhelmed with the information he had given me. I remember crying at that appointment too because again he confirmed what I didn't want to hear. Even though I knew that it was wishful thinking, I was hoping that I'd meet with him and he'd tell me that it was all a mistake. That after conducting their own scans, they noticed that it was a benign tumor. For the first two weeks after being diagnosed, I was full of tears, but I knew it was ok to get it out before I started my fight. Once I started my fight, I told myself that I wouldn't cry. I now know that it's not safe to think that way, but it was the way that I needed to think in order to make it through the storm successfully. Please anyone going through the storm, cry if need be. What worked for me may not work for you. This path will be different for everybody going through it. I only hope that some of the things that I went through helps you.

He also knew about my mother and her illness, so he had to know how emotional this appointment was for me. He assured me that everything would be ok. After telling me that someone would be calling me to have the chemo port put in, we scheduled my first chemo appointment for the Friday after next and my chemo teach class for the following week. We ended the appointment with a prayer. Having an oncologist who believed in prayer and spoke about God directing his path was the most calming part of that appointment. Being diagnosed with breast cancer is one of the hardest things that I've ever had to endure, but I felt at peace knowing that I was doing it with someone who had a strong faith level like mine. I prayed to God for me to find a medical team that I had favor with, and I felt assured that he had answered my prayers by sending me my medical team.

After meeting with the doctor, I got a tour of the facility. Most importantly, the infusion room. The infusion room is where everyone sits and have their chemo treatment. Although I pretended that I wasn't bothered, it was hard to see the room full of chairs with IV bags hanging from ports next to it. Most if not all of the patients wore hats, scarves, or showed their natural bald head. I knew this would be my fate within the coming weeks but to see it first hand was another gut punch. I had to remember that HE wouldn't bring me to it if he wasn't going to bring me through it.

I called my mother and sister immediately after that appointment upbeat. Even though I was getting ready to fight one of the hardest fights in my life, I felt good. I knew that I had what I needed to make it through. I was excited to tell my mother about my oncologist and his faith level. I was happy to tell her how he ended the appointment in prayer. My mother was happy to hear it. She was always a firm believer in making each move with faith involved.

Chemo Teach Class

I debated going to this appointment. If I attended the class that meant that I was accepting my diagnosis and everything that I would have to endure in the following months. If I didn't go, I could continue to deny the inevitable until I couldn't. Not knowing what this class would consist of was the hardest part. I didn't know if I'd go to a class with a ton of people that were scheduled for chemo or if it would be a one on one appointment, but I knew that going was the right thing to do. So I took my first step in being a fighter and attended the class. When I got to the appointment, I sat with the nurse practitioner only instead of being in a class full. She gave me a book that she said would answer any questions I may have. The book included everything that I needed to know in order to be my strongest while enduring chemo treatments. The book explained the types of chemo I'd be taking along with the medicines that I would be prescribed, when, and how often to take them. That appointment was my first real step in the fight.

> **Reflecting back to my mother's battle** - When I think of my chemo teach class, I think of my mom. A couple of days after I went to this class I was told by my mother that she had decided to take a couple of rounds of chemo. I remember sitting in a chair in her bedroom following my class and her telling me that she had decided to give it a shot at going a couple of rounds. She told me that she would be taking the class and starting her treatments around the same time that I would be starting my treatments. Of course, she made sure to let me know that her starting treatment did not mean that she didn't believe. For some reason, I think she thought that if she accepted any form of treatment, it meant that she didn't believe in God's will. I hope not because I accepted treatment, but I still believed that God was and would always be in control.
>
> My sister accompanied my mother to her chemo teach class. I was excited to know that I would be going through one of the hardest ordeals in my life

with my biggest supporter. No, I wasn't happy that either of us had to endure this but who better to endure it with. While my mother did attend the chemo teach class, she never got the chance to start the treatments. She was hospitalized shortly after and became too weak for treatment.

The Big Chop - September 16, 2017

I knew that I would lose my hair courtesy of the chemo treatments so I wanted to take destiny in my own hands by cutting it down so that when it did begin falling out it wouldn't be as emotional. I heard horror stories about people losing globs of hair after a couple of rounds of chemo treatments and how hard it was emotional to see it. I didn't want to be one of those people.

I remember my sister being really emotional when she started losing her hair after having a couple rounds of chemo treatments. She would talk about having globs of hair on her pillow and in the shower. She often told us how hard it was to see. She was the first person that I knew of to cut her hair to save herself from the emotional roller-coaster when it began falling out. One morning after waking up and seeing hair on her pillow, she decided that she would no longer let the superficial things slow her from her mission of healing. That morning she decided to shave her hair. I was so shocked that she would just shave her hair. I remember thinking that I would hold on to my hair for as long as I could. Now after going through the same journey, I understand. I know that her shaving her hair was a brave thing to do. At that time, she cared less about her appearance and more about her emotional state. I know this because I went through the same thing.

There were several women on videos that I watched the night that I was diagnosed who also talked about cutting their hair. I knew then that I would do the same thing when the time came. I knew that there would be so many things that I would have to endure during this battle so I wanted to control the things that I could so I cut my bob length hair into a pixie cut the week before my first chemo treatment. Thank God the short pixie cut fit my face or I would have felt horrible. Instead, I felt in control. My beautician and I talked about my hair cut as if I was getting it done because I wanted something new. She knew about my diagnosis and the reasoning for doing so, but I am sure she was taking my lead. Because I talked about my storm as something that I was going through but would soon come out of so did she. There was an older lady there who listened to us talk, and that was shocked to hear why I was getting my hair cut. Before leaving the room, she told me that she would be praying for me and that meant a lot. I'm a firm believer in there being power in prayer, so I welcomed prayer from anyone.

I walked into my sister's house after my hair cut and received compliments from my family about how good the cut looked on me. My uncles were there at the time because they were in town checking on my mother. I saw a look of both sadness and proudness on their faces. I told them that I was scheduled for my first chemo appointment on Friday and cutting my hair was my first step in accepting and fighting my condition all at the same time. This was hard to accept, but I knew accepting it was the only way for me to stay upbeat and positive while doing so.

When I walked into my mother's room, I saw a proud look on her face. She told me that she liked my cut and that she knew that I would be ok. Being diagnosed wasn't ideal for either of us, but we both knew that we had the fight within us to beat it. I'm sure cutting my hair confirmed what she had told my sisters when she found out that I was diagnosed. She told them that she knew I was going to be ok because I knew God and my faith level was strong, and because of it I was a strong woman. Even though what she said may have been true, I was a little unsure if I had what it took to make it through this storm because I was unsure of what the storm entailed.

Port Installed - September 19, 2017

The day that I was scheduled to have my port installed, I was extremely nervous. I was the girl who had to be carried to the dental and doctor's chairs kicking and screaming when I was younger preparing to have a procedure that involved needles, and I had no say so about it. I needed the port installed in order to receive my chemo treatments. I was both nervous and scared but I knew I had no choice so again, I had to put my big girl panties on to make it through.

I was told not to be scared because I would be sleep during the procedure. WRONG! Once I was in the back and prepped for the surgery, I was told that I wouldn't be put to sleep, but I would be drugged good enough so that I wouldn't feel anything. "IS THERE SUCH A THING!" I thank my husband who was there and knew how frightened I was for putting my mind at ease. Because we both are extra goofy, we were able to laugh when others would have cried, and it actually worked to relax my nerves. No matter how hard he tried, he failed at hiding the fact that he was nervous as well. I caught him gazing into space a couple of times, which is something he does when he has a lot on his mind. I understood the feeling though because I did too.

Thank God my port was successfully installed, the bad part is that it was 2 days before my first chemo appointment which meant that it would probably still be sore when it came to getting my treatment.

1st Chemo Appointment - September 22, 2017

The morning of my first appointment I was extremely nervous. With all of the stories that I'd heard about chemo treatments, I didn't know what to expect, and that was scary. My biggest concern was that I would become nauseous and throw up everywhere. Another fear that I had was that my veins would explode once the chemo started flowing through. I was even afraid that whatever was getting ready to start flowing through my body would make me stop breathing. I was given some lidocaine cream and was told to heavily coat the area where my port was installed on the day of my appointment. The lidocaine cream was supposed to numb that area. I made sure to put an extra coat on before leaving home. I thank God that I was able to stay positive and instead of being sad and crying I smiled and laughed the entire way to my appointment. I even sent my family a picture of me with my lidocaine cream covered by saran wrap. No matter how I felt about what I was getting ready to do, I knew I had to do it, so there was no reason to be down or depressed about it.

When I first arrived at the oncology office, I was told that I was scheduled for labs, to see my doctor, and then the infusion room for treatment.

Lab

The first time that I had to give blood I was petrified. I squirmed the entire time and also reached out with one hand to pull the nurses hand back so that she couldn't insert the needle. I knew that I had to get used to needles because I would have to endure them every other week for the next several months. I did not conquer that fear at my first visit.

Infusion Room

After labs and meeting with my oncologist, I stood in the infusion room where I would receive my chemo treatments for the next couple of months. Both my sister and husband were at this appointment. I remember us looking around at 20 or more chairs that were stacked around the room with a pole for the IV that would hold all the meds that I would be receiving from the port that was just put in two days before. Being in that room was very emotional for me because it was at that meeting that I was in the same predicament as the 60 and 70-year-old patients that had been blessed to live a full life. I could no longer deny that I had cancer and that I needed to receive chemo treatments in order to become a survivor. In my 30's all I ever thought I would have to worry about was raising my children while working on advancing my career but it was evident that God had other plans in store for me.

After introducing myself to the nursing staff, I was told to sit at the seat of my preference and someone would be there to assist me. When the nurse came to connect my port to an IV, I experienced the worse pain of my life. I had applied the lidocaine as instructed, and it was pointless because the incision and the area where my port installed was still tender and sore. The purpose of the lidocaine was to numb the skin so that I wouldn't feel the stick. I don't know if it was because of the swelling or that the lidocaine just didn't work, but I definitely felt the stick. When the needle pierced through my skin to connect to the port, I teared up. It took two nurses to connect my port to the IV.

While I wanted to leave and say forget it, I knew I couldn't because like my husband said, if I wanted to be a breast cancer survivor I would have to endure it and since becoming a breast cancer survivor was my mission I stayed. Thank God they were able to hook everything up so I could receive my first dose of chemo.

Chemo Treatments

I received three different chemo meds that day. The red devil was one and I was told that it was a concoction of two meds. Halfway through my chemo appointment, a nurse came around and attached what she called the Neulasta onto my belly. She explained that the purpose of the Neulasta was to help my body make white blood cells after receiving chemo. Within a minute of when she stuck it to my stomach, I felt the light sting to the stomach. The worse part of the whole process was the suspense of wondering when the sting would happen. She told me that I would receive the medicine through the plastic needle that was inserted inside my stomach at least 25 hours later. I remember hearing the beeping noise the following day letting me know that the medication was starting to run through my body.

I was given the Lupron shot that day as well. The purpose of the Lupron shot was to suppress my hormones. Because my cancer was hormone-based, it was very important to suppress them.

Cancer treatments have progressed a lot within the last five years. My sister had to go back to the facility the following day to receive her Neulasta shot. Five years later, I was able to get mine by sticking a device to my stomach and receiving the medication the following day. This proves the importance of research and donations to conduct those researches.

My Mother

I remember going to see my mother the day after my first chemo appointment. She was laying in the bed at my sister's house. I was shocked when I walked in to see that her hair was missing in the front. Because she was receiving radiation treatments for her head, the hair in that area fell out. She also had a black mark on her forehead, but I had no idea why. Again, looking at her in that state sent me into a panic because not only did I worry about my mother, I felt like I was getting a glimpse into my future.

I couldn't let her know that I was worried so I pretended to act normal. I'm sure she knew that I was bothered because she was good at reading me. We talked about my first chemo treatment. She asked me how I felt after taking it and if I was still happy that I decided to take treatments. At this point, she was still against chemo treatments, so I knew that I needed to tread lightly when discussing it with her. I told her that I was feeling fine and I was still happy that I decided to have the treatment. I told her that as long as God gave me the strength to do so, then I would continue to do so. While she was able to decide to forgo treatment, I couldn't. All of my mother's kids were adults but I was still raising mine. I knew I had to give this fight all that I had so that I could look into my kids face if the time comes and tell them that I did all that I could do to beat this disease and be here for them.

We went on to talk about the type of surgery that I decided I would have and why. I told her that I would be having a double mastectomy when the time came. Again, I wanted to do all that I could do. On top of being opposed to having any type of chemo treatments, she was opposed to having any body part removed, so she was against a mastectomy or lumpectomy. She respected my decision but reiterated that none of the things that I was doing to beat cancer were for her. I felt horrible hearing that. I loved my mother and confided in her about everything, but I knew that in order for me to win this battle I would have to discuss it with someone who felt like the step that I was taking was the right one.

How I felt following my first chemo appointment

I immediately picked my children up from aftercare following my first chemo appointment, and we went to my niece's tennis game. My way of thinking was that I wasn't going to let the chemo prevent me from doing anything unless I didn't have the energy to do so and since I had the energy to make it to the game, I did. I shockingly had the energy to sit through her entire game. I imagined that my chemo treatment would be a lot worse than it turned out to be. I thought immediately after my appointment I would get nauseous and throw up everywhere right before crashing. Thank God I didn't.

The first couple of days after receiving the chemo treatment, I was fine. By the third day, the draining feeling that I had heard so much about was setting in. I was almost finished with my steroid and anti-nausea medication, so I didn't have any pain or nausea issues so I thought I would be fine going back to work by the fourth day after chemo, but I was wrong. My commute to work was an hour with traffic, and by the time I made it to work, I was drained. I was able to make it through that day and half of the next but decided then that starting with the next treatment I would be working part-time and that I would take the week following chemo off. That was the only way that I would be able to be my best, and I wanted to give my employer my best.

Not only was I tired throughout the day but I couldn't sleep well throughout the night. Between the hot flashes and hunger caused by the steroids, I either woke up in night sweats or felt like I was on the verge of starving to death.

Unfortunately, I was tired up until the next treatment, so I struggled to work consistently. Things that I was not prepared for was happening to me, like when the chemo had my head feeling cloudy. This is when the "chemo brain" started. Chemo brain is what my sister called forgetfulness. I never knew how real it was until I experienced it myself. It's like I was so tired that my brain was unable to process the things that I normally did so I had delayed responses. This also included me forgetting things. The big wall calendar that I had bought several months before had become my best friend. I had to jot down everything on that calendar. This included: all of our monthly bills, doctors' appointments, kids' events, and anything else that it was imperative for me to make it to.

Prescriptions

The medications that I took following my first treatment was Claritin, Dexamethasone, and Zofran for nausea to take as needed. I was told that the Claritin and Dexamethasone were both for the aching and swelling in my bones. The Zofran was for nausea. This was on top of the Zofran that I was given in my IV as part of my treatment.

Side Effects

The side effects that I experienced were: weakness, hot flashes, slightly lightheaded, and my stomach felt weird like it was feeling up with something. I had no idea what that something was. I slept throughout the days for the first week. Thank God that my husband was able to be there for the kids because I was of no help. I didn't experience the emotional side effects that my sister did or the nausea side effects that many others have, but I endured fatique that I would've never imagined possible if I hadn't experienced it myself.

Chapter 2 - Second Chemo Appointment - October 6, 2017

My second round of chemo treatment went off without a hitch. My husband and I sat around for at least 4 hours while the poison was once again being injected into my body through the port. By that appointment, we had realized that we had an emotional journey ahead of us with the chemo treatments, and the best way to make it through was to treat the chemo appointments like a normal appointment, so we brought snacks, worked on the laptops, played games on our phones, and talked about everyday dealings during that time. A nurse came around while I was receiving the chemo and attached the Neulasta on my stomach.

I remember looking at the other patients with either their scarves, hats, or bald head. My hair did not fall out after my first treatment so I thought I would defy the odds and wouldn't lose my hair. I decided that even if I did, I would wear either a hat or a wig to my chemo treatments.

By this treatment, I was still working, but I was now on a part-time basis. Unfortunately, I hadn't been working at my job long enough to take any temporary leaves, and I knew working as a paralegal for a small firm that they would need someone to be there full-time. I hated to make the decision, but I knew that I would soon have to resign from my position. I talked to the office manager who asked me to stay long enough to train my replacement. I told her that I would which meant my last day would be at least 3 weeks away.

Hair Falling Out Like Crazy

A week after my second round of treatment is when my hair started falling out like crazy. Unfortunately, I did not defy the odds. I too would have to live without my hair for several months. Knowing that it was a possibility and actually having it happen are two different things. Going through losing my hair at 36 was rough. I was never a big hair person but not having the option to have it was a blow to my ego. I didn't have time to get used to my hair falling out because when it started, I began losing hair everywhere.

I was losing hair in places that I didn't even realize I had hair. There were times when I would be lying in bed and out of instinct I would run my fingers through my hair, and I would pull back a clump of hair in my hand. My shower was clogged with hairs that I didn't even realize were falling out. Little did I know, my husband had noticed the hair in the drains before I did. Because he didn't know how I would react, he never said anything about it. He said he felt better waiting for me to broach the subject. Losing my hair was very dramatic for me, but I couldn't let it derail me from my mission of making it through the storm. To this day, when I run my fingers through my hair, I have a nervous feeling in the pit of my stomach that I will pull back a clump of hair.

October 16, 2017 - The Shave

After begging my brother to cut my hair and him telling me no, I decided to do it myself. My brother and I have always been close, so I understood that cutting my hair may have been too emotional for him, so I didn't want to push him to do something that he wasn't comfortable with.

I had a cousin in town the weekend that I decided that I was going to shave my hair. She and her mother were in town to check on my mother. My cousin and I were at my sister's house sitting on the couch talking when I told them that I was going to cut my hair. Our children were also in the room talking to each other. They both gave me a look of shock over wanting to shave my hair. While my cousin raved about how inspiring it was, my sister was stuck in her feelings which were obvious by the watery look in her eyes. I'm sure it was hard for her to imagine seeing me with no hair. After explaining the many reasons why I had to shave my hair, I told them that I didn't want to wait any longer because I wanted to do it then and now. Emotionally, I was tired of running my fingers through my hair and pulling down clumps of hair but more than anything I knew that doing so was starting to affect my son. It seemed like he was around every time I touched my hair and pulled away with clumps. When he saw it, he'd get sad and ask me to stop touching it. In his little mind, he believed that if I stopped touching my hair, it would stop coming out.

I begged my sister to help me shave it, but she was very emotional. I completely understand that it was hard hearing that I was diagnosed. I remember how hard it was several years prior to when we heard those words from my sister. Also hearing those words from my mother's doctor was hard. Even though she acts like she wasn't, my sister was still having a hard time accepting my diagnosis. When she became teary-eyed, I knew that it was too much pressure for her so I told her that I would do it myself hoping once she saw how positive I was about shaving my hair she'd be ok. To dry up her tears and keep her from breaking down into a fit of tears, I joked back and forth about my hair coming out in clumps. In my family, we learned to deal with pain by laughing instead of crying whenever possible. I knew that she needed to laugh, so I began pulling small clumps of my hair from my head and blowing it in her direction. That made her go from sadness to humor. She eventually began laughing, and we went into her bathroom where I planned to make the cut.

I used her husband's clippers to start my bald cut. I started cutting my hair from front to back. There was no reason to be strategic with it because at the end the plan was for it all to be gone. I cracked jokes about it the entire time by making buzzing noises while cutting. We were going through enough as a family.

My mother was at my other sister's house in the bed where she had been for days. She'd started complaining about headaches, dizziness, and blurry vision. I knew that's where our focus needed to be, so I refused to use any of our energy on me when I was fine.

After cutting front to back a couple of times and messing my hair up a lot, my cousin joked about how bad of a job that I was doing before grabbing the clippers and cutting the sides. My sister then grabbed the clippers and finished the back. Before we knew it, we all were taking part in shaving my hair. I didn't care how it came off; I just wanted it off.

When I walked out of the bathroom, and my son saw my bald head he instantly cried. I don't know why not but I wasn't prepared for his response. I hate that I didn't prepare him beforehand. I was so busy worrying about taking the pain away from him by cutting my hair that I didn't think about how that would affect him to see me go from my hair falling out to completely gone.

My advice to anyone going through this with children, please involve them in the process so it won't be so hard for them to accept. If I could do this over, I would have let my husband, son, and daughter help me with this cut.

Mom was checked into the Hospital - October 19, 2017

My mom was checked into the hospital again. This time it was for not drinking, eating, and she started losing focus. She seemed somewhat incoherent. I hated that she was being checked in, but I wasn't shocked. My siblings were all at her house a couple days earlier trying to get her to eat. For the second time, we were struggling to get her to go to the hospital where she would receive the best care. She was both drained and didn't have an appetite.

I remember my siblings and I working on a welcome home video for my sister who is an airman in the military because she was coming home from overseas. We all were in the front room working on the videos while my mother was in the back laying in her bed. I remember hearing her constantly going back and forth to the bathroom and hearing her throw up before going back to lay in her bed. She did this several times that night. While my sisters kept saying she was ok and that she was throwing up because of a virus that she caught from my son who was sick the day before, I knew it was more. I was stressed over her health that entire night, but I tried hard to leave it in God's hand.

I remember my sister texting me that night and asking me if I thought that the headaches and dizziness could be caused by the cancer spreading to her brain. I told her yes, because prior to her texting me I was on the internet conducting research for her symptoms and brain cancer was the main cause of it.

I decided not to go visit my mother the night that she was checked into the hospital because it also happened to be the night before my 3rd chemo treatment. I needed to keep my mind strong to continue to fight my battle and seeing my mom laying in the bed in so much pain would definitely weaken me. It sucked because I felt that I was at a point where I had to choose myself over my mother. I was afraid her time on this earth was limited, and I wanted to spend as much time with her as possible. How unfair to be going through what I was going through and not only was I having to do it without my biggest supporter but I wasn't able to support her when she needed me most.

How I felt following my second chemo appointment

Like the prior treatment, this treatment was fine. The third day was when I felt a change. Thank God I didn't have to deal with the nausea that I heard others complain about. My main issue was my strength. I was so tired. All I wanted to do was lay around, which wasn't an option because I was still working and my children needed to get back and forth to school when my husband was at work. I was able to eat, but unfortunately, nothing I ate was fulfilling because my taste buds were off. I no longer had an interest in soda and coffee because of the taste. Some of my food selections had changed as well. I began eating for sustenance instead of enjoyment.

The week after my treatment, I dealt with constipation. While I was lucky enough not to have to deal with hunger problems, I had issues with drinking enough water. I was never a big water drinker, so it was even worse now that I was being made to drink it. I was afraid of ending up like my mother or other patients who suffered from dehydration because of their lack of liquid. I would do everything that I could to get fluids. I started eating Jello and sucking down popsicles on the regular.

Prescriptions

For the three days following chemo, I took Dexamethasone, Claritin, and Zofran as needed.

Side Effects

The side effects that I experienced following my second treatment were weakness, horrible hot flashes, slight lightheaded, and constipation. I just wanted to sleep for days.

Chapter 3 - Third Chemo Treatment - October 20, 2017

I sat at my third chemo appointment receiving my treatment through my port, and all I was able to think about was my mother's dwindling health. I wondered what predicament she would be in if she decided to take chemo. While I kept saying to myself that she wouldn't be in the position that she was, I knew that was a lie because God had her where he wanted her. On the way to him. I constantly prayed for her and stayed in contact with my siblings during my treatment to stay updated on her condition.

My treatment went good that day. I tried hard to treat it like any other visit and thank God it was. The lab went better than it did the time before. The phlebotomist was able to find a vein. My sister told me that when she was going through chemo, she had problems with them getting blood. She was told that the chemo was burning her veins. I don't know how true that was, but I definitely had issues when trying to have blood drawn.

My appointment lasted a little over 3 hours. During my treatment, it felt like every time I sat in my chair I was up dragging my pole to the restroom because of all the water I drank.

The nurse put the Neulasta shot onto my stomach that appointment as well. My family and I finished that day off by going to the movies. Thank God I was in a position to sit still and watch the whole thing without going to sleep. It was very important for me to keep things as normal as possible for my kids because I felt like the last year of their lives were sad and depressing. Following my mom's medical scare, she was moved to Texas from Illinois where we lived to receive care. On a daily basis, my children were able to spend time with my mother at a nursing home that she was staying at right up the street from us.

My kids went from seeing her daily to seeing her on a weekly basis when she moved 30 miles away to stay with my sister. Because of the pain that she was in, she was then checked into the hospital where they hardly got the chance to see her. I hated it for my children because not only were they watching me going through chemo and battling cancer, they were watching their grandma lose her battle with cancer.

It was almost a week after I received my treatment before I was able to go visit my mother in the hospital. I barely had the energy to walk from my bed to the couch daily for the first week. Thank God for family because I was no help to her. A few of my mother's siblings took turns coming in town staying for weeks at a time to help care for her. My 96-year-old grandmother even stayed weeks at a time to be with my mother. I will never be able to express how much they being there for us helped and how much we appreciated it. Most of my siblings lived out of state. The ones that lived in the area where my mother was hospitalized worked full-time, so they were unable to help as much as needed. I wasn't much help myself. I worked part-time, and when I wasn't working, I was sleeping trying to recuperate from my treatment. During those days is when the guilt and sadness began setting in. I felt guilty because I was not in a position to help the lady who always had my back for my 36 years on this earth when she needed me most. I was sad because I knew we were living in her last days so it was now or never so there were days where I was totally exhausted, but I would push myself to get up just so I could go put my eyes on her. By now she was in and out of consciousness, and when she was conscious, I'm not sure she knew who I was. Imagine being by your mother's bedside and seeing her in so much pain and there is nothing that you can do to help her. Take it a step further and imagine your mother looking up at you from her bedside and you know that she has no idea who you are. That was me. When I looked into my mother's eyes, I saw something different. I couldn't tell if it was a look of worry, fear, pain, or just a look of tiredness. I was dealing with all of that while going through one of the hardest times of my life.

At times I felt that when she looked at me, she pretended that she was ok when it was evident that she wasn't. There my mother laid in bed in pain, but she acted otherwise to protect me. She knew how much it hurt me to see her in pain knowing that there was nothing that I could do. Gone was my vibrant fast-talking mother who would playfully threaten her children with sayings like, "We are going to fight and I ain't gonna lose" or the woman who would send us text messages like, "CP" and we were supposed to know that she meant "cold pop" or "Pepsi" to be precise. Most importantly, gone was the person that I would turn to when I needed her and I needed her now. I wanted to talk to her about how big a deal my hair loss was because I knew she would have the right thing to say. Because of my hair loss, I had to take on the burden of choosing who was strong enough to see me bald without emotionally breaking. There were days that I would have friends and family come over and I would have to either wear a wig or cap so that they were ok. My mother was the person I wanted to discuss my struggles with being so drained while keeping it together for my family. She knew how important it was for me to take care of my family and because of my energy level, I was unable. She was also the person who I wanted to discuss how hard it was to watch my mother dying right before my eyes and that it was being caused by the same illness that I was fighting. I was so overwhelmed with everything going on. Again, I was in a place to remember that God put me in a place to remember that HE should've always been the one that I leaned on to discuss everything and because I didn't I was lost. I had to accept the reality that my mother was just loaned to me and he was rescinding that loan.

Check-up with my Breast Specialist/Surgeon

I knew that I would have to see my breast specialist while going through chemo. She told me that she would be periodically seeing me to check the progress of my tumor. My first appointment after I started chemo I was nervous, and I had no idea what to expect. After pleasantries, she conducted an ultrasound of my tumor. I heard her slight inhale before asking her assistant to hand her an instrument that she used to check the size of my tumor then she asked her the original size of my tumor. Her assistant looked in the computer and quickly confirmed the original size of my tumor. Hearing all of this back and forth between them had me worried that I was getting ready to hear more bad news when my doctor turned to me and told me that I could sit up and she went on to tell me the best news. She said that according to the size of the tumor on the screen, my tumor had drastically shrunk. She went on to talk about how shocked she was to see it shrink so much so fast. After asking the normal questions (How was I feeling, any new issues, etc.), she told me that her office would schedule an appointment with me to see her again in a few months.

We walked out of the doctor's office feeling so good that day. I couldn't wait to pick my kids up from school so that I could share the good news with them. So far, they'd been doing well with the physical and emotional changes that I was going through. I remember when I first shaved my hair, I would wear hats and scarves around the house so that they wouldn't be emotional every time they saw me. Shockingly, they took it better than I thought they would so I stopped wearing anything while at home. They would rub my bald head daily and tell me how soft my skin was. I was never a touchy-feely person, but I knew that this is what they needed to be ok with what was going on, so I let them touch away. I was so happy to see that my kids were learning to roll with the punches that life was throwing us.

My children are different, so I had to look extra hard when it came to making sure they were doing ok emotionally. While my son is very emotional and wears his emotions on his sleeves, my daughter does not.

My son was scared to leave my side because he was afraid that if he did, I wouldn't be there when he came back. My daughter who is more of a watcher would watch me from afar and ask a ton of questions that I was happy to answer. To ensure they were ok, I knew I had to be strong while fighting this battle. I knew there would be times where I would be in pain but that I would have to downplay it for my kids' sake. I also knew that there would be times where I was drained and would want to sleep for days, but I would have to get up to show them that I was ok. I also knew that there were days when I knew I would want to cry and give up, but I knew that I couldn't. I knew a lot of things would go on over the next several months that I had no control over, but I knew that I had to be in control of those things, so I prepared to do a lot of smiling when I wanted to cry.

I was scared about how my diagnosis and journey would negatively affect their lives. Things were, in fact, turning out better than what I thought. When we picked the kids up that day and told them that my tumor was shrinking, they both got so excited, and my daughter even said a prayer to God thanking him. The journey that I worried about negatively affecting my kids was bringing them closer to God. We've always taught them about God and prayer but going through this journey they were able to see God's work. I knew that this journey wasn't going to be easy, but as long as there was a purpose in my pain, I was cool.

The news from the doctor was exactly what I needed to hear. My mother's health was steadily going in the wrong direction, and it was draining on me emotionally, so the good news was great.

My mother slipped into a coma

My mother went from sitting up in the bed staring at whomever came to visit her pretending like she knew who they were, to slipping into a coma. The last couple of visits I spent with her, she stared off into space like she was talking to someone that I couldn't see. On one hand, I prayed that she was talking to the Lord, but on the other hand, I knew that if she was that meant that her days on this earth were numbered.

One day I walked into her room thinking I'd be able to talk to her knowing that she wouldn't respond when I was told that she was asleep and had been for a while. I still visited her constantly after she slipped into the coma, but instead of talking to her I'd talk to whichever family member that was sitting with her about her health.

Because I had started my chemo treatments, I was constantly being told that I shouldn't be at the hospital because of my risk of infection. My options were that I could either risk my health but be able to spend some time with my mother or stay away from her and miss out on the chance of ever seeing her again. I was filled with so much pain and anger about having to make that decision but I couldn't pity myself over what I was going through. I felt that doing so would only make me weak and I needed to be strong if I wanted to make it through the storm.

My life consisted of going from chemo appointments to the hospital to sit next to my dying mother's bedside. That had become my reality.

How I felt following my third chemo appointment

Like the prior treatment, this treatment was fine. The third day was when I felt a change. Thank God I still hadn't had to deal with the dreaded nausea that I heard others complain about. My main issue was still my strength. I knew to get everything that I would need for days 3-6 before my chemo treatment because it would be an issue to get out and get anything afterword. I was still on my one week half a day scheduled. Although I wanted to, I was unable to give my employer any more of my time. By this treatment, I was drained longer than I was the other times. I was unable to fully recover from my last chemo appointment before having to endure it again. This meant that I was tired at work and my energy was almost depleted by the time I made it home. I decided that I could either split my energy between my family and my job or give it all to my family. I decided to give my all to my family. I resigned effective the first week of November. My appetite was still good, but my taste buds were still off, so I continued eating my Jello, popsicles, apple juice, fruit punch (Hey I had to get any type of fluids possible and drinking water was becoming a hassle). Because of the steroid, I had a fourth meal time. Middle of the night! I would wake up in the middle of the night and eat either a sandwich or a Lunchable along with a drink. My mother was given steroid medication by her doctor when she moved to Texas. I remember her waking up in the middle of the night when she stayed at my house to eat. I used to laugh at her thinking that she was just hungry. She would tell me that her appetite was due to the steroid. Now I understood exactly what she meant.

Prescriptions

For the three days following chemo, I took Dexamethasone, Claritin, and Zofran as needed.

Side Effects

I experienced the same side effects: weakness, horrible hot flashes, slight lightheaded, and constipation. I just wanted to sleep for days.

Chapter 4 - Fourth Chemo Treatment - November 3, 2017

I was getting ready to walk out of the door for my fourth chemo appointment when I received a call from my older sister. She told me that she received the results of her biopsy. There was a spot on her MRI report that she took the day with me and they wanted her to go in to have a biopsy done on her breast. We both knew that she would get a negative result, so we weren't too bothered. Again, I thought there was no way that God would allow our family to get hit again when he knew that we were struggling with the first two cancer diagnosis. The wind was knocked out of me when she told me that the results were positive. My heart stopped beating for a few seconds. All I could think about was that our family was being hit with another person being diagnosed with breast cancer.

I had two emotions going through me as I took in the news. One was sadness that my sister and her family had to go through this and the other consisted of a fighter mentality. "If he did it before he could do it again" is all I could think because I knew that the same God who healed my sister years ago and who was directing my steps to ensure I was a survivor was the same God who would ensure that my sister would also be a survivor. For weeks after I found out that I was diagnosed I wondered about God's purpose, now I felt like I knew. Even though I hated it, I realized that God was getting ready to call my mom home and the purpose of my sister and me being diagnosed was to give my family something else to focus on when we lost the matriarch of our family.

When my sister called and told me about her diagnosis, she told me to stay quiet about it until she had a chance to speak with her family. The night that I was diagnosed, I decided to sit my children down and tell them about my diagnosis. As expected, they cried which broke my heart. The most important thing to me was for them to be ok and I knew that they needed to hear that I was ok for that to happen. I wanted them to know that even though we'd be going through some hard days, we would all be partners in this. That worked for my family. I completely understood my sister wanting to talk to her family about it before letting everyone else know.

Unfortunately, my sister was unable to get the same vote of confidence from my mother about her being strong enough to make it through her storm. My mom was in a coma when we got the news that my sister was diagnosed, so she never got the chance to talk to her about her diagnosis. I'm not sure it would have mattered if she was told because when she slipped into a coma she was a completely different person. I'm not even sure she would've been able to receive the news.

My younger sister and brother were both at my house at the time that I found out. I knew that it would be hard to talk to them and not tell them about the horrible news that I was just told but I knew that I had no other choice.

We talked about them wanting to accompany me to my chemo appointment, but because of the 1 guest per patient rule at the facility, they wouldn't be able to. They would be made to sit in the waiting room for 3-4 hours and I didn't want them to have to do that when they could be sitting with my mother. My husband had accompanied me to all of my treatments up until that point. It was easier to go through each of my appointments with him because there was no pressure for me to be strong. Because we were used to what was happening behind the doors of the infusion room, it wasn't as emotional to us as it once was. I knew that my sister and brother would be emotional if they were to come back and see me receiving my chemo treatments and that would make me weak. They decided that they still wanted to come and would wait in the waiting room until they were ready to go to the hospital to be with my mother. I guess being near helped them emotionally cope. I understood that because I did the same thing by visiting my mother who didn't know I was there. Again, I saw my battle being a testimony for my family.

Good News

With everything that was going on, I was happy to get the good news from my oncologist that I would only have to do 4 more rounds of chemo instead of the 8 I expected. He told me that I would continue to take my treatments every other Friday instead of the every Friday that I expected. "Thank you Jesus" is all I could say. I was so thankful to be almost done. Thus far, none of the scary things that I heard of had happened so I heavily prayed to God that they wouldn't. I remember coming to my first visit with my oncologist and being told by one of his nurses that there was a strong possibility that I would have to do 8 more rounds following this visit and those treatments would be weekly. I was so happy that her prediction was wrong. I was told by my doctor that the results of my genetic testing dictated how many more rounds he would recommend and since my results came back negative I only needed 4 more rounds. He also said that my remaining four treatments would be of Taxol and not the three types of chemo that I had previously taken.

He tried putting my mind at ease by telling me that most people said the Taxol was easier than the chemo that I had previously taken. This gave me hope that everything would be ok. Thus far, I hadn't had any major issues with the chemo. Just mostly fatigue.

My mother's health continued to decline

When my mom was first diagnosed, my family and I couldn't fathom losing her. We were still not ready to lose her several months later, but we knew it was a possibility. We went from having a healthy mother to one who was on her deathbed and having doctors telling us that any day that we had with her was a blessing because they didn't expect her to live long.

According to the doctors who originally diagnosed her with cancer 9 months prior, the tubes that they inserted in her would never be removed. They even doubted that she would ever leave the hospital. We as a family were happy that not only did she leave the hospital she was well enough to move 13 hours away, had the ventilator and all the tubes that were running through her removed, she regained her ability to talk, she went from a wheelchair to a walking stick to walking on her own. There was even a time after she moved to Texas that she came over to my house and played basketball with my daughter, nephew, and me. I knew that the time we got to spend with her after she moved to Texas was a blessing so instead of focusing on her health I focused on the memories that I was able to make with her. I appreciated the blessing that we received from God when he spared her life giving us several months with her following her diagnosis.

I hate that my sister was unable to get that vote of confidence about being strong enough to make it through her storm from my mom that I did. My mom was still in a coma when we got the news that my sister was diagnosed, so my sister was unable to talk to her about her diagnosis. I'm not sure it would have mattered if she was told because when my mother slipped into a coma, she was no longer the person I knew, and she probably wouldn't have been able to receive the news.

Emotional state following my sister's appointment

I remember sitting with my sister at her appointment with the same breast specialist that told me that I was diagnosed with breast cancer. Unfortunately, my sister would be hearing those same words from her. My sister would also be given a treatment plan to beat cancer's butt. I knew how emotional this appointment was for me, so I knew that she had to be feeling emotional as well.

I thought back to sitting in this waiting room for the first time. I spent it people watching. I looked to gauge the ages of the patients that came and went. I wanted to know their ages because at 36 I felt too young to have to deal with this. I also looked to see if the patients wore a defeated expression or not. I wanted to know how they were dealing with their diagnosis.

As I sat and waited with my sister, I thought back to the young African-American couple that couldn't have been that much older than my husband and me that came in the office that day. I watched as they discussed how many cancer treatments she had already endured and how many she had left. As I looked on, I realized that they didn't seem defeated. Instead, they looked like fighters who were treating a cancer diagnosis like nothing more than an obstacle that they had to overcome. I wish I could see that couple again and thank them because watching them I realized that I too had the strength to fight too. Watching them gave me that "if they can do it we can do it" attitude so I knew then that if I received the dreaded news that I'd been running from for over a year, that my husband and I would endure the same fight to win.

After waiting in the waiting room for over an hour, my sister, her friend, and I sat in one of the patient rooms listening to the doctor give my sister her prognosis which happened to be a lot different than mine. The doctor gave my sister different treatment options that she could take in order to beat cancer. This was a lot different from mine because I was given commands that I had to follow in order to beat it. I was so happy that her news was better than mine because the life that I was living and the worry that came with it was not fun. Hearing the doctor talk to her about her prognosis and her treatment plan that was different from mine also was another reminder of how bad of a situation that I was in and how hard my fight would be. I prayed to God to give me the strength.

Tamara B. Newborn

My Mother Flatlined

A few days after my sister's appointment my mom flatlined. My sister sent us a text message through our group chat telling us to get to the hospital as fast as we could because our mother had flat lined. She said she wasn't sure if she would make it until we made it, but we all took off running hoping that she would be ok.

I remember getting off the elevator on my mother's hospital floor and looking into the glossy eyes of my sister, brother, and cousin who were at the hospital with my mother. As I walked down the hall towards my mother's room, I saw doctors and nurses running in and out of it. My sister told me that she was talking to my mother like she normally did when my mother began gasping for air and all of her monitors started beeping. She said when she asked the nurses and doctors for help they swarmed in the room and asked them to wait outside. My sister talked about how scary it was to be there when everything was going on, and I knew it had to be very hard. To be honest, I'm not sure I would have been strong enough to see it because emotionally I was a wreck.

I know that it would have made an already weak me dismantle to be present when my mother was gasping for air and hearing all of the machines going off would have made things worse. I was told by my sister that it took a few doctors and several nurses to work on my mother, but they finally found a pulse. She was resuscitated and rushed to the ICU on the 2nd floor.

We stood outside of my mom's hospital room on the second floor watching the number of doctors and nurses swiftly going in and out of her room. My sister was telling me how close to death my mother had come when I looked up in time to see my aunt swiftly walking down the hallway towards us. My sister had also called her when my mother was being resuscitated. My two aunts and grandmother were all staying across the street the entire time my mother was in the hospital. Thanks to Reba Ranch House it was at no cost. I was able to see the sadness and panic in my aunt's face as she walked towards us to get an update on my mother's condition. She was huffing and trying to catch her breath. It seemed as if she ran over when she got the news. After giving her an update letting her knew that they were able to resuscitate my mother, my aunt released a breath of air that she'd been holding. The entire walk or should I say run over, it had to be going through her head that my mother would have taken her last breath before she arrived.

Up until that point and time, my aunt was able to act unfazed over what was going on with my mother. We all knew that she and the rest of my mother's sisters were hurting over slowly losing their sister. My mother and three of her sisters that had been rotating in to help us care for her for weeks at a time were all within an age or two together so they went through almost everything in life together and I knew that it had to be hard on them to be losing her. They sat back for the last couple of months of her life and watched their sister transition out of this world and did it with a brave face because they knew that's what we needed to stay strong and I thank them so much for that. Seeing them crack would have definitely made me crack more than I already was.

I spent the next several hours at the hospital that day thinking about how close I was to losing my mother. I knew this meant that my mother's condition was a lot worse, so I needed to prepare myself for the inevitable. This was the point where I was having the internal back and forth about believing and accepting. I knew as a family; we needed to accept that we had some decisions to make.

On top of all of the emotional struggles we had to endure with my mother and her condition, we also had to battle with her medical staff over her medical care. Unfortunately, the doctors began pressuring my family about signing a DNR (Do Not Resuscitate) for my mother. They continued telling us that she was living in her last days and that she wouldn't recover, so there was no purpose in prolonging the inevitable. I remember a doctor telling us that she would probably crash again that day, the next day, or a week later but he said it would be soon. He said us not signing the DNR was only causing more harm on her body, but all we could think about was honoring my mother's wishes of fighting until she had no fight left. Signing the DNR was going against everything she fought for. Considering how adamant my mom was about fighting to live we felt it was only right that we continued to fight for her as well so we told the doctors that we would not sign the DNR.

For the next several weeks we were constantly harassed by the medical staff to sign the DNR. There was also a time where they slid the paperwork in with other papers my sisters had to sign on my mother's behalf hoping she would sign it instead. I thought it was weird that they were so passionate about us signing the DNR when she hadn't had any issues since she was moved to the ICU. Either way, it was hard to hear them say over and over that we needed to forget the possibility of her bouncing back as she did before.

I didn't want to lose my mother especially when I needed her most, but more importantly, I didn't want my mother to suffer, and I wasn't sure that she wasn't. I had come to a point where I was emotionally drained, and when I wasn't resting, I was worrying about my family. I worried about my mother in her state. I worried about my father who was losing his wife of over 40 years and who had to be strong for his kids' sake. I worried for my sister who was served the biggest blow by being diagnosed with the same illness that my mother and I had, but because of everything that was going on with my mother, she had no time to focus on herself and mentally prepare for her new reality. By this point, my sister had to accept the fact that she would have to fight this battle without the bid of confidence that we craved from my mother, because it was highly unlikely that she would be able to give it to her. I was starting to accept the fact that my mother was living on borrowed time, while most of my siblings thought that there was still a chance that she could make a comeback like she did several months back.

How I felt following my fourth chemo appointment

Like the prior treatment, I was fine after taking this treatment. I had my normal sore throat the day after my treatment, and I'd noticed a couple of sores in the inside of my mouth. I gargled with the recommended salt mix when I remembered or had the energy to do so. The third day is when I felt my biggest bout of fatigue. Thank God I still had no nausea issues, but my energy level was still low. I had finally resigned my position at work, so I no longer had to pull myself up to go to work for my half day week, but I was spending more time at the hospital with my mother.

Thank God I was able to spend the times when I did have energy with my family. My appetite was still good, and my taste buds were still off, so I was just eating for sustenance and not for enjoyment. I continued eating my Jello, popsicles and drinking water as much as possible.

Prescriptions

For the three days following chemo, I took Dexamethasone, Claritin, and Zofran as needed.

Side Effects

I experienced the same side effects: low energy and horrible hot flashes.

Chapter 5 - Fifth Chemo Treatment - November 17, 2017

I began my treatment of Taxol this visit. I was extremely nervous because I didn't know what to expect. The nurse told me that Taxol would be a lot easier than the chemo that I'd previously been taking but that she had patients complain about tinkling in their fingers and toes. She also said that I might notice a change in color in my nailbeds. She said ice might help slow down the effects, so she recommended that I bring icepacks to my appointment just in case I needed it. It sounded embarrassing, so I decided that bringing bags of ice was something that I wouldn't do. I decided that I would see how this appointment went and if I needed the ice, I would bring the ice to my remaining visits.

My doctor, his nurses, and others that I researched said that the Taxol treatments would be easy, but that didn't put my mind at ease. I was nervous that with this treatment I would start to have some of the complications that I had heard about but had yet experienced. My biggest concern was that I'd be nauseous.

It was at this appointment that I met my friend J who I stayed in contact with for the remainder of our treatments. I remember her because she was there with her mother who had bags of ice that she packed on her hands and feet. While it was a little strange to see, I wasn't totally surprised because of what the nurse told me. Seeing them together always made me think of my mother who instead of being with me while I had my treatments was laying in a hospital bed fighting for her life. I always worried while taking my treatment that I'd get that call saying my mother had passed away. It was so hard to concentrate on the here and now because my mind was always with my mother. I didn't want my first treatment of the new meds to turn out bad, so I laid back while the Benadryl ran through my system.

There was a flood in Houston before this appointment, and because of it, there was a shortage of IV bags. Starting that appointment, I received most of my preventive meds (steroid, nausea medication, and Benadryl) by being pushed through a syringe instead of the IV bags that I had become used to. This way was actually easier.

Neuropathy

I remember reading people say they used the cooling treatment to prevent nail issues. They complained about Neuropathy which I later found out is a nerve damage that is caused by the Taxol treatments. I was told that if this occurred that I would feel a burning or numbing feeling in my hands, feet, or both. Seeing my friend with the ice bags had me thinking that maybe I should have taken the treatment to prevent neuropathy more serious.

Because I didn't follow the same ice treatment that my friend did, the tingling started following my first appointment. It wasn't really painful, but it was uncomfortable, and my fingers felt tight. My fingernails eventually turned either all black while my toenails were white. I had white spots in my toenail and in my fingernails I had black spots. My sister scared me away from getting pedicures because of the potential of an infection. I'd paint them myself when I had the energy and had my daughter do it when I didn't.

I was told that I wouldn't have to take the steroid after my treatments with the Taxol because it wasn't necessary. Again, I was told that most people didn't need the steroids because the treatments were not as harsh. Unfortunately for me, I felt the worse aching of my whole treatment when I didn't take any steroids after this appointment. I remember sitting in my mother's hospital room with my sister and father and complaining the whole time about how bad my legs were aching. I was tired like normal, but the aching was overweighing my lack of energy. When I called my doctor's office and complained about the aching pain, I was given a prescription to restart the steroids. Unfortunately, the chemo that was easy for everyone wasn't going to be so easy for me.

My Mother began slipping away

By my fifth chemo appointment, my mother was still in the coma that she had fell into a month prior. I would walk in and out of her room without her knowing that I was there. At times, I would just stand back and watch her. I was too afraid to touch her because I was scared that I'd break as soon as I did and I knew I had to stay strong in order to make it through chemo. Her eyes would fly open when we would sit in the room and talk which in the beginning we took as a sign that she was looking at us. We later found out that it was not the case. I grasped everything that she did as a sign that she was still with us when I knew in my heart that she wasn't. It was evident by the way her pupils looked when her lids popped open that she wasn't looking at anything in particular.

My poor mother had lost a ton of weight so going into her room and seeing her tiny body lying in the bed was so hard. The hospital did a great job of moving her around every so often, but she was still starting to have bed sores. I was happy that my mother wasn't suffering, but I selfishly wanted her here with us. I wanted her healthy and well, but I was coming to grips that she was transitioning to be with the Lord. Watching my mom dwindling away and having to be ok with it was one of the hardest times of my life.

The doctors were still pressuring us to sign the DNR, and now on top of that, they were asking for permission to take my mom off the machines. It was their opinion that she was gone and us continuing to let her live on the machine was cruel. I began stressing about if I was cruel by continuing to let her stay on the machine in hopes that she came out of the coma and healed up to become the person that she once was or was it cruel to take her off the machine and take away any fighting chance that she may have. When my mother first got sick, she told us that she wanted to fight and I wondered if taking her off of the machine was taking her option to fight.

After dropping my kids off at school in the morning, I would go sit with my mother until it was time to pick them up and either my sister or my aunt and grandma would come sit with her until someone relieved them later that day. I sat with her on Monday and Tuesday of that week. I came in and sat by her bedside typing on my computer while her lifeless body laid still on her bed. The entire time that I was there, her body made no movement. The only noise in the room came from the machines and me tapping the buttons on my computer.

My husband came that Tuesday. It had been almost a week since he last saw her, but he expected for her to look the same. Unfortunate for him, she didn't. She had lost more weight, her eyes were sunken in, and her complexion was darker than it was before. Her entire appearance was different. I could tell that it was then that he realized the end was near for her. We both looked over at each other with the same look of acceptance.

I was ready to admit it to myself that continuously coming to see my mom in the state that she was in was eating me up. It was beginning to throw me into a depression, and I couldn't allow that because I needed to stay strong in order to take my 6th chemo treatment the following Friday. For some reason, I just knew that my mother was gone.

Thanksgiving 2017

This was by far one of the worse thanksgivings that I've ever experienced. It didn't feel like a day of celebration but more like just another day. My mother had been in her coma for over a month and her condition was worsening. My family rotated in and out of the hospital that day to make sure we spent time with our mother and our families. My family normally got together at one sibling's house annually but this year was different. We all ate at our separate homes. We all were emotionally, physically and mentally drained. Our mom was the person we called a million times during the holiday to ask recipe questions. We had all just dealt with the first holiday not being able to do so. Knowing that Thanksgiving was one of our mother's favorite holiday we knew that she would not want to be laying in a bed, but instead, she would love to be at my sister's house eating with all of us.

It was so horrible to have her living so close to us but not with us. It wasn't fair that she was laying in the bed slipping away instead of celebrating the day with her family.

How I felt following my fifth chemo appointment

Like the prior treatment, this treatment was fine. The third day was when I felt a change. Thank God I still hadn't had to deal with the dreaded nausea that I heard others complain about. My main issue was still my strength. My appetite was still the same. My taste buds were off, so I ate for sustenance and not enjoyment. It was still hard for me to drink as much water as I needed, so I continued eating my Jello, popsicles, and drinking water as much as possible.

Prescriptions

For the three days following chemo, I took Dexamethasone, Claritin, and Zofran as needed.

Side Effects

I experienced the same side effects: weakness, horrible hot flashes, slight lightheaded, and constipation. I just wanted to sleep for days.

Chapter 6 - Sixth Chemo Treatment - December 1, 2017

When I went to have my sixth chemo treatment which entailed my second dosage of Taxol all I could think about was my mother. Between my mother's dwindling health and my fear about taking Taxol, I didn't have a good feeling when I went to that appointment. By this treatment, my mother had been in a coma for over a month, and her health was continuing to get worse. The doctors repeatedly told us that there was nothing more they could do and begged us to take her off the machine. I was constantly praying for her to make a miraculous recovery even though I knew the likelihood of that was slim to none. To say I was stressed over her condition was an understatement because by this appointment I had accepted that my mother was transitioning out of this world. I remember the last time I'd seen her which happened to be two days before my chemo appointment. She didn't look like someone who was still living but instead she looked like someone who was existing, and that was thanks to the machine. I felt that my mother was no longer on her way out of this world, but instead, she was already gone. I feared that my father, siblings, and I needed to discuss funeral arrangements, but because they were keeping the faith and believing that she would recover, I was scared to share my belief. My faith level was as strong as everyone else's, but I just felt that God was calling her home.

On top of worrying about my mother, I was still nervous about my body having a bad reaction to taking the Taxol, and I soon found out that I was right. Unlike the first dosage of Taxol and all of my previous appointments, I had complications while receiving this treatment. I was an hour into my treatment when I began having back spasms that were almost unbearable. My heartbeat sped up, and it became difficult for me to breath. I was afraid that this was it. This treatment would be the cause of my death. I was going through some pain and shortness of breath that I'd never before endured. My husband and mother in law both accompanied me to this appointment, so I got my husband's attention and asked him to get my nurse quick. He was shocked that I was having issues because it was a first so instead of running for the nurse he asked me a million questions. My mother-in-law who realized the urgency told him to hurry and get help. When my nurse came over, she gave me medications that stopped the pain, and she slowed down my dosage.

Before starting this treatment, I was told by my medical staff that my Taxol treatments wouldn't take as long as my previous treatments took because the drug would be given to me at a quicker pace. After my bad reaction to receiving my treatment quickly, my nurse told me to tell the nurses at all my remaining appointments that they needed to give me my medication at a slower pace. She told me that for some reason, my body was having a bad reaction to the medicine when given at a fast pace. That fear that I had about taking Taxol was creeping back in. I was also angry. I had made it this far without any real complications, and because of this bad reaction, I now dreaded my remaining two chemo appointments. I feared that the next time the nurse wouldn't be able to slow down the treatment and the pain would be a whole lot worse or possibly fatal. I began feeling like I was the low percentage girl. If there was a low percentage of a reaction, it would happen to me. All I could think was "Lord please don't let this stop me from completing my full treatment of chemo." I was on a mission to beat cancer and I couldn't stop even if I had one of the hardest chemo appointments ever.

GOODBYE MOTHER – December 1, 2017

I received a call from my sister at 4:20 pm today telling me that my mother had passed away. After not being able to get us to sign the DNR giving them permission to take her off the machines, they told us that if any of her scans ever came back with no brain activity, they had the legal right to take her off the machine. The scans that they conducted that day came back saying that my mother had no brain activity. The inevitable was happening and there was nothing that we could do to stop it. The fight was no longer hers or ours to fight. I prayed to God to accept that everything was according to his plan.

The doctors told us that they would keep her on the machine for a couple more days to give family the option to come see her. Even though I hated getting that phone call, I wasn't shocked because I knew that she was gone when I last saw her. It did suck knowing that I only had a couple days to see my mother and then she would be gone forever. This meant that I would soon become one of the motherless children of the world. That inner strength that I'd been leaning on for the last several months was becoming weak. I knew I had to make it, but I didn't know how I could. On top of everything that I was going through with my chemo treatments and my physical strength, losing my mother was a big blow. Inside I knew that she wasn't going to make that miraculous recovery, but there was always still a little ounce of hope. I prayed harder than I'd ever prayed that night. I knew that I couldn't bring her back, but I prayed to God to give me the strength to live without her.

My mother was in a coma for at least a month and a half before she passed, so I wasn't able to have a two-way conversation with her, but I was able to talk to her and pretend that she was listening. I knew my mother well enough to know what advice she would give me about what I was going through, so I didn't need to hear her response. Even though she was unable to respond, I still felt like she was listening. I had no choice but to accept that I would no longer be able to have a mother/daughter talk. The person who I talked on the phone with 2 maybe 3 times a day was gone. I had no one to talk to about that, and it sucked. I was going through so much, and the person who I would normally talk to about it was no longer an option. It sucked to be fighting a battle against cancer but having to do it without my biggest supporter because she was losing her battle to cancer. During those days, I talked to God and told him everything that I wanted to tell my mother.

My mother-in-law happened to be at my house on the day that I got word that my mother had passed. It was the evening after one of my chemo treatments. I thought back to the talk that my mother-in-law and I had a couple hours earlier about my mother. I told her how much it bothered me to have my mother's body lying in her hospital bed plugged up to the machine when I was almost 100% sure she was gone. My mother-in-law told me that I didn't have to worry about making a decision because God would handle it. I remember us sitting at the table and having a discussion about my mom's condition. I told her how much it bothered me to have my mother's body lying in a hospital bed plugged up to a machine when I was almost 100% sure she was gone. I was in turmoil about her body being removed from the machines. By this time, I was sure that she was transitioning out of this world. I knew that the dream that my family had about her recovering like she did before was just that, a dream. My faith level was as strong as everyone else's. I felt like everything happened in accordance with God's plan and I felt like God was planning to call her home.

My mother-in-law told me that I didn't have to worry about making a decision because God would handle it. Not even an hour later, I got a call from my sister telling me that the doctors had declared my mother brain dead. They said that they would be giving my family a few days to come say goodbye before taking her off the machine. I was in turmoil about her body being removed from the machines because that meant that she would be forever gone, but I knew they had to. I wanted to cry and crumple over knowing that my mother was leaving me, but my mother-in-law wouldn't let me.

Two days later, my sisters and I sat down to discuss the steps that we needed to take on our mother's behalf. The plan was for my sisters to go to the hospital after our meeting and give the hospital permission to have my mother removed from the machines. Emotionally, I was super weak and knew that this was something that I needed to take a step back and let my sisters handle. Physically, I was drained from the treatment that I had two days prior. During our meeting, we cried and laughed as we discussed the wonderful memories of my mother and information about her home going celebration. That was by far, one of the hardest things I ever had to discuss and while going through one of the hardest times of my life.

After our meeting, my sisters went to the hospital to have my mother removed from the machine. Soon after, I got a call from them letting me know that she stopped breathing within minutes of being unattached from the machine and that the doctor had officially pronounced her dead on December 3, 2017.

A few days later my sisters and I flew to our hometown where we would be laying my mother to rest. Even though we were all sad and somewhat hopeless, we tried to be strong as possible as we worked together to get it all done. We worked on pure adrenaline because that's all we had. The matriarch of our family was officially gone. We had no idea how we would make it without her, but we knew we had no other choice.

Thank God for family because our family was so supportive through this whole ordeal. They stepped in to do the things that we were too weak to do. We had family who prepared my mother's makeup, family who made sure everything was ready at the church for the funeral, the same thing for the gravesite and the family that helped for my mother's repass. It was a comforting feeling to see my family bond together when we all needed each other. My mom had touched a lot of lives, so there were plenty of people who wanted to step in and bet a part of her home going celebration.

Being with our family had us laughing when others would have been crying. It was so good to be back in the folds of our family, but we knew that it would soon end. We all had to go home and when we did our new reality would begin. For me, it was accepting the fact that I would have to learn to live without my mother. I wouldn't ever see the words "mom" come across my cellphone screen. I wouldn't be able to say "mom" in a direct conversation. My life had changed drastically, but I had no time to dwell on that reality. Thank God for our faith level. Leaning on God was the only way that I was able to make it through that week. I was so busy worrying about my sister and my chemo appointment that I didn't have time to dwell on how much pain I was in from losing my mother. When I caught myself falling into a depression where I wanted to cry I would pull myself out by thinking about what all I still had to accomplish in order to win my fight. I missed my mother like everyone else did, but I was unable to mourn her like the rest of my family. While they had the luxury of falling and getting up I didn't. "A weak person would have issues making it through chemo," I thought and I had to make it through. I pushed myself during this time harder than I ever had. Even though no one admitted it, I know that I was constantly being watched by my family to make sure that I was ok. I was super close to my mother and when she passed, I continued living life like nothing had happened. I wouldn't even allow myself to cry. I know they were afraid that I would have a meltdown and I couldn't tell them that I wouldn't, all I could tell them was to catch me if I did. I hoped that smiling when I was sad and diverting my mind would all keep me from doing so. Plus, I was taking my mother's passing a lot better than I thought I would have. I thank God for my faith because I know that's the only way that I was able to make it through that storm.

Our travel home after burying my mother was the longest drive I've ever taken. Everyone was gone, and now I had no choice but to accept what I was going through. During the 16 hour trip home that normally took 13 hours, I had nothing but time to think. It sucked because when I got home, my mother would no longer be there. I wouldn't be able to go see her at the nursing home, I wouldn't be able to see her at my sister's house nor would I be able to see her in the hospital. Now if I wanted to see her, I'd have to visit her at her gravesite 13 hours away and even then I wouldn't be able to look into her loving eyes. I'd be talking to her headstone. I was hurting so bad while accepting this new reality but I knew I had no other choice but to accept it. I was going through a storm that I knew wouldn't last forever but making it through it was so hard that I knew I'd come out with war wounds to show.

While I love my mother and I will always miss her I try to look at the positives like she didn't suffer in her last days because she slipped from a coma to death. I knew that where she was going, she would never suffer again. I took solace in believing that while she wasn't cured on earth, she would be healthy and happy where she was going.

How I felt following my sixth chemo appointment

I was scared to come to this appointment because I didn't know what to expect. I never expected to have the reaction that I did, but after slowing down the drip, I didn't have any other issues. My appetite was still good, but my taste buds were still off, so I continued eating my Jello, popsicles and drinking water as much as possible.

Prescriptions

For the three days following chemo, I took Dexamethasone, Claritin, and Zofran as needed. On the recommendation from my doctor's office, I purchased vitamin B and L-Glutamine that were supposed to help with the tingling and tightness in my fingertips.

Side Effects

I experienced the same side effects: weakness, horrible hot flashes, nails were still turning colors, and I had the tingling in my fingers.

Chapter 7 - Seventh Chemo Treatment - December 15, 2017

Almost a week after burying my mother I sat at the bedside of another loved one. My sister was in recovery after enduring an 8-hour double mastectomy. By the time I made it to the hospital for my sister's surgery that morning, she had already gone back, but I sat with her family in the waiting room. Because I had to take my kids to school that morning, I missed her because she was already in the back when I arrived. Her husband and daughters told me about how high her spirits were when she went back. While the normal person would have been unable to make it for that surgery, she accepted the challenge. Not only did my sister have to bury her mother a few days prior but this surgery was scheduled a few days after her 40th birthday. I was filled with so much pride at seeing my sister being the fighter that she always was even though I knew it had to be hard on her because it was hard on me and I wasn't the person having the surgery. I thank God for equipping us with the strength necessary to make it through our storms because they were coming back to back.

I left halfway through her surgery for my chemo appointment. I dreaded this appointment more than any of my other ones. I was afraid that I would have another reaction and I was afraid that it wouldn't be as easy to reverse the symptoms. My mind was going crazy with everything that I was going through, and I was afraid that if I did have another reaction, I wouldn't live to tell the story. I remember talking about my mother to J and her mother at that appointment. They wanted to know how she was doing, and they were shocked when I told them that she had passed and I had just come back from burying her days before. I remember the looks they gave me. They were full of sympathy, confusion, and surprise. In their heads, I'm sure they were thinking that I should be acting a lot different than what I was, being that I had just lost my mother. Yes, I was deeply hurting inside, but I knew that I couldn't let that pain crumple me, so I didn't. I prayed to God for strength and understanding that she was in a better place.

The neuropathy was still a factor, but the tingling and pain were bearable especially when I had bigger things to worry about. Thank God that the appointment went as smoothly as the others had. The whole visit including my labs, meeting with my doctor, and actual treatment lasted about 4 and a half hours. They slowed my drip when giving me my treatment and that helped a lot. Throughout that treatment, all I could think about was my sister and her surgery. I guess having my mind occupied helped my time go by faster, but it did nothing for me mentally because I was a wreck.

When I returned to the hospital to see my sister a few hours later, I was told that she was still back in surgery. Nine hours after she went back we were able to see her. My sister's family, her in-laws, and half of my siblings were there when she came out. After all of the emotional crap that my sister had been through, I thank God that she made it through this surgery like a champ.

3 Day Hospital Stay

After spending the Christmas holiday with my younger sister and her family, I came back to town to visit my older sister who was still in the hospital. She was originally told that she would be released from the hospital 5 days after her surgery and here it was going on day 12 so I was really concerned. Unfortunately, my sister had to spend Christmas in the hospital. Thankful that her family was able to celebrate it by decorating her room and exchanging gifts in her hospital room. By watching them, I learned that we can either allow our storms to make us or break us and her family definitely used this storm to make them stronger.

We were eventually told that my sister had developed an infection and that was the cause of her fever and pain. The infection that she had was uncommon. She was told that she would have to have a small procedure to correct the issue. I was unemployed, but my sister's husband wasn't. He had been staying at the hospital the entire time that she was there which meant that he was missing work. My sister repeatedly told him that she would be fine and for him to return to work. I'm sure he was worried about his wife staying alone. I knew how that felt because that's the same way we all felt when it came to my mother and her hospital stay. I told him to go ahead and go to work the following day, and I would be there to spend the day with my sister. I knew I needed to rest because I was exhausted and having breathing issues, but I knew that if I were to stay home, I wouldn't get rest anyway because I would worry about my sister the entire time. I also ignored my couple of episodes of sharp chest pains that I had experienced at my younger sister's house. While there I experienced my biggest bout of drainage. I was so weak that all I wanted to do was sleep.

When I got up the following morning, I was experiencing the same draining feeling that I had suffered the past few days, but I shook it off like normal exhaustion from my chemo treatment. I still had the shortness of breath, and now my heartbeat was beating faster than normal, but I couldn't let my sister sit at the hospital alone, so I pulled myself up. Because my mother was gone, I felt like I needed to be there in her place.

My sister had been told the night before that she would be having a small procedure that day and I wanted to be there when she went back this time. Thinking that no one was at the hospital with her besides her teenage daughter, I knew I had to be there.

When I got to the hospital the following morning and made it to my sister's room, I saw a room full of family. Through blurred vision and shortness of breath I struggled to walk to the couch but I knew I needed the rest. My heart was beating faster than it had been when I walked from the garage to the hospital elevator minutes earlier. By the time I fell onto the couch I could hardly breathe, and it was evident by my watery eyes and constant coughing that I was having problems breathing. I didn't know if my condition was caused by the chemo that I was taking, my exhaustion, or the pneumonia that I had self-diagnosed myself with. What I did know was that I needed to see a doctor to get medicine before my condition worsened.

While we waited for them to take my sister back for her procedure, I laid on the couch that was sitting in the corner of her room. I knew I couldn't do anything that would cause me to become weaker. When my sister went back, I decided that I would go to the emergency room and get medicine since I knew it would be a couple of hours before she'd be done. I thought that I would go to the emergency room and tell them my issues. After they ran several tests, they would give me medicine and I'd be back in my sister's room before she was. Unfortunately, that wasn't the case. An hour after checking into the emergency room, I was calling my husband at work to tell him that I was being checked into the hospital for an overnight stay. All I could tell him was that they were checking me in for heart problems because that's all I knew.

The admitting doctor told me that he was uncertain about my heart condition, but he was worried that I had a heart attack sometime before coming to the hospital. I thought back to the heart spasms that I had while at my younger sister's house for Christmas. I didn't pay it any attention; because I thought the spasms were just a side effect from the chemo. The doctor wanted me to be checked into the hospital where the nurses could keep an eye on me while I waited to see a cardiologist who would be making his rounds the following day.

After taking several different EKGs, I was told by the cardiologist that I didn't suffer from a heart attack but Broken

Heart Syndrome instead. He said that my body was having a reaction from all of the stress and suffering that I had endured the previous months. I remember him saying to me that even thought I wasn't grieving my mother's passing and dealing with all of the stress that I endured since being diagnosed didn't mean that it wasn't happening. He said my body took on the stress and was the cause of my heart problems. The way he explained it was that Broken Heart Syndrome is stress induced and that it is caused when the body goes through stress like I had been through. He said that the symptoms are similar to having a heart attack but nowhere near as severe. I was happy to hear that it wasn't a heart attack. With everything that was going on, the last thing that I needed was to have to worry about another illness.

I stayed hooked up to the heart monitor the entire time that I was a patient. My heartbeat was too fast, and this affected my blood pressure. They took several tests to make sure that everything with my heart was fine. All tests came back good with no issues, so they were never able to explain the issue with my blood pressure and heartbeat. I was given a heart medication when I was released. My heart issue worked itself out when I was released.

When I was checked in, my family was again worrying about two people. Instead of it being my mother and me like before, it was now my sister and me. Thank God that my sister's persuasive skills were great because she was able to persuade her medical staff to give her a couple of hours to come and see me. Our rooms were directly one floor apart. When I came back from one of my scans, she was sitting in my room. I was so happy to see her because I was worried about her. She looked so good which meant I didn't have to worry about her. Seeing her sitting up and looking healthy after having surgery a couple of days prior gave me the strength to keep it moving. If she was capable of being on the move after what she'd been through, I knew I could be strong enough to make it through this obstacle.

I was by far the worst patient because I constantly complained about being released. My vitals were high, and I had a slight fever so they wouldn't release me. I didn't know what it would take for everything to be fine, but I knew it had to hurry and happen because I had my last chemo appointment scheduled within a couple of days and I didn't want to miss it. I was sad to be told that I wouldn't be able to have my chemo treatment if I still had my fever. Unfortunately, I still had a fever, and because of that and the fact that I was still checked into the hospital, I missed my 8th and final chemo appointment. This meant that I had to reschedule my last treatment for some day within the new year which would stop me from accomplishing my goal of completing chemo in 2017. I found myself being halted by another bump in the road that prevented me from obtaining my goal of beating cancer. Little did I know that this wouldn't be the only time that things wouldn't go as I expected.

What I learned from this whole ordeal is instead of stressing and being sad when something doesn't go as I expect, accept that there is a reason and that I don't need to know it. Also, I learned that things wouldn't go as I wanted them to but as God wanted and it would happen in God's speed. I thanked him for the things that did go my way and prayed for me to accept the things that didn't. Because of the curveball that I was being thrown, I had to achieve a whole new level of patience.

After begging and pleading with the medical staff, I was released from the hospital after three days, and it also happened to be the day before New Year's. Even better was that my sister was also released that day.

Thank God because my siblings who had just buried their mother a few weeks earlier were running from the cancer floor to the heart floor to visit my sister and me. That time was so stressful for my family, but with the grace of God we made it through.

How I felt following my seventh chemo appointment

Thank God that I didn't have any problems with this treatment. I still had the tingling in my fingers, and more of my nails were turning black. When I could remember, I was still taking the vitamins that were recommended by my doctor's office that were supposed to help with the tingling. My appetite was still good, but my taste buds were still off, so I continued eating my Jello, popsicles and drinking water as much as possible.

Prescriptions

For the three days following chemo, I took Dexamethasone, Claritin, and Zofran as needed.

Side Effects

I experienced the same side effects: weakness, horrible hot flashes, fingernails were still black, and my toenails were white.

Chapter 8 - Eighth and Final Treatment - January 5, 2018

I had my eighth and final chemo treatment 3 days before my 37th birthday. Everything went good that appointment including the Labs. They were able to take my blood with no problem. I spoke to my doctor who gave me the results of my blood tests which were all good. We set up an appointment for me to come see him after my surgery. He said we would discuss the next steps then. I assumed that the next steps would entail us discussing a hormone blocking medication like the one that my sister was taking. I later found out that I was wrong. I had my last chemo treatments in the infusion room and thankfully everything went smoothly as well.

I didn't know about the big celebratory bell that everyone rings on the last day of their chemo treatments, so I didn't ring it at the end of my appointment. I was so excited about being done that I nearly sprinted out of the office that day. It felt so good knowing that I had accomplished a major goal in beating cancer by completing chemo. I was so excited because this was my first step on the way to being cancer free.

I reached out to J who was scheduled to have her surgery within the next week. She told me about a mass that the doctor had found in her breast. She said they weren't sure if the mass was cancerous or not so she would have to take another MRI. She promised to update me as soon as she could. Hearing that she possibly still had cancer in her breast wasn't a shock because I was told that the chemo was given to me before surgery in hopes of the lump decreasing but I didn't take that to mean that the cancer would be gone. I spoke to her again a few days later, and she told me that the doctors saw something concerning on her records so they decided to move her surgery up. We made plans to talk again after her surgery. I prayed for her to have a successful surgery and speedy recovery. We both were fighting hard to be survivors. We did everything that was asked of us in hopes of being survivors.

Prescriptions

For the three days following chemo, I took Dexamethasone, Claritin, and Zofran as needed.

Side Effects

I experienced the same side effects: weakness, horrible hot flashes, fingernails were still black, and my toenails were white.

Pre-Surgery Appointment

I saw my breast specialist prior to my surgery that was scheduled on my sister's birthday of January 23rd. She told me that it was possible that my surgery would have to be pushed back to a later date because my chemo was completed late. She explained that there needed to be a certain amount of days in between chemo and the surgery and that she wasn't sure that I made the cutoff. She told me that she would have to check with the other doctors and that she would let me know. Again another possible roadblock on the road to becoming a survivor. All I could do was silently pray that God would handle this issue like He had handled each one before.

In the meantime, my doctor discussed my surgery as if I was going to have it as previously scheduled. She told me that she would perform the first half of my surgery and my plastic surgeon would perform the second half. I was told that she would remove both of my breasts and some of my lymph nodes to check for cancer. She said that while the tumor had decreased significantly, it was still there. I was told that my plastic surgeon would insert expanders in the space of my breast tissue. The expanders would be used as a space holder so that my skin didn't heal while I endured radiation. I was told that I would have to see my doctor for several visits after that surgery to have the expanders pumped with fluid.

For the next couple of weeks while I prepared for my surgery, I prayed over and over again that my surgery would be a success.

I MUST!

Matthew 17:20 (KJV) *– And Jesus said unto them, Because of your unbelief: for verily I say unto you, if ye have faith as a grain of mustard seed, ye shall say unto this mountain, Remove hence to yonder place; and it shall remove; and nothing shall be impossible unto you.*

Chapter 9 -Double Mastectomy - January 23, 2018

The day before my scheduled surgery, I had to see a cardiovascular doctor to get the clearance for the surgery. I was told by my oncologist that he wanted to ensure that my heart was strong enough to endure the surgery. There was something that the ER doctor put in my discharge papers that gave him concern. I was given the ok from the cardio doctor the day before my surgery. Knowing that my surgery was a go brought about all types of feelings inside. I was happy that the time had finally come where I was knocking down another speedbump on the way to becoming a breast cancer survivor. I was scared about what would happen during the surgery. I was told about the procedure that would be performed on my lymph nodes and for some reason that was the scariest part. The procedure consisted of injecting a liquid in my breast using a needle. Like I previously stated, I have a fear of needles, so I was halfway to an anxiety attack by the morning of the surgery. I was sad that again I was going through something in my life when I needed my mom, and unfortunately, she was no longer there for me to give me her words of support or her strong prayers that always left me feeling like I could beat whatever obstacle it was that I was fighting. Because I no longer had my mother to lean on, I had to make it my business to lean on the Lord. I did what had become my norm since being diagnosed and prayed to God for strength.

My in-laws came in town the night before my surgery to ensure that they were able to be with my husband and me on the day of surgery. I thank God for their support because I knew I didn't have to worry about my husband with his family around. I was prone to worrying, and I tend to worry even when there is no reason to. Needless to say, I did a lot of worrying while going through this storm.

When I woke up the following morning my heart was heavy. I wasn't as nervous as I thought I'd be, but I was sad. I was missing my mother a lot. My family walked around the house that morning like it was a normal day when inside we knew it wasn't. After dropping the kids off my husband, father in law, mother in law, brother-in-law and I walked into the hospital where I would walk out a few days later without breast. It sucked to know that I would be missing one of the main things that made me a woman but I couldn't dwell on that fact.

I was in my hospital gown and lying in my hospital bed within 30 minutes of arriving at the hospital. My sisters and brothers arrived shortly after. Once again, I looked into their eyes and was able to see the pain that was present last year when my mother, sister, and I were diagnosed. I don't know if seeing me in my hospital gown in the bed preparing for surgery made them scared that I would end up in the same place as my mother, but I definitely saw worry in their eyes.

Lymph Node Procedure

My brothers came in one by one with a look of fear in their eyes. I understood that they were nervous about the surgery, but my mind was elsewhere. While most people dreaded the double mastectomy, I dreaded the injection that I was getting prior to my lymph node removal surgery. My sister who had it done a month ago wouldn't tell me exactly what would happen, but the way she looked when I asked about it made me feel like it wouldn't be good. I was wheeled back to the radiology department where the injection would take place with a mind full. While I waited in the back on the radiologist who was in seeing another patient, I almost had an anxiety attack. I even considered getting up and making a run for it, but I knew that I couldn't have the surgery without this procedure.

The radiologist eventually came in and performed the procedure. The way he explained it was that he would be injecting a radioactive substance around my nipple that will help the surgeon find and remove the lymph nodes. He couldn't tell me how my lymph nodes would be removed, but he told me that the purpose was to see if they were still cancerous and that there was a way for them to know the likelihood that the cancer spread outside of the node. I thank God because the procedure was nowhere near what I imagined. I think the only pain that I felt was the pain that was caused when he injected the numbing medicine. After that point, I didn't feel anything. I was eager to get back to my room so that I could tell my sister how wrong she was for having me afraid for no reason.

I was wheeled back for my surgery almost immediately after getting back from the lymph node procedure.

Recovery from Double Mastectomy

I remember being wheeled into my room after my surgery and thanking God for coming out. My family was already there in the room. The doctors updated us on my condition and left the nurses to take care of everything else. I was given the morphine push that I was able to push every time I felt pain. That, and the fact that I was still numb, I didn't feel a lot of pain. There were times when my blood pressure was up and my heartbeat was fast, but the nurses watched it so that it didn't become a big issue. The heart issue was the same thing that I experienced in December that there was no medical reason for. Following the lymph node procedure, I was very uncomfortable. I felt like my underarm was carved out and that made it hard for me to lay in certain positions. The next several days went well, and I was able to be released on time.

Tamara B. Newborn

Chapter 10 - Post Operation Appointment with my Breast Specialist

My sister came to town a week after I had my double mastectomy. She wanted to be around to take me to my post-operation appointments. I remember her saying, "since mom is no longer here, I feel like it's my responsibility to be." I hate that she put all of that pressure on herself, but I love her for doing so because I really needed her. My mother had passed a little over a month before, and my sister knew how emotional I was even if I didn't show it.

My sister accompanied my husband and me to my post operation appointment. The doctor came in and reviewed my pathology report. I was so nervous to hear what she had to say. She told me that at the time of my surgery, my cancer had shrunk drastically but that I still had a cancerous tumor in my body. She also said that they removed 6 lymph nodes from my body and 1 of the 6 still had cancer. She went on to say a lot of other things, but I have no idea what they were. I zoned out! While the doctor was talking, all I could think about was that I still had cancer. I felt like everything that I went through the months prior was for nothing. I hated it but I knew that I would have to endure everything that I'd been through the previous months because I still had cancer in my body and I wouldn't rest until it was all gone.

I'm sure my sister was able to look into my eyes and see both sadness and panic there because she quickly interrupted the doctor. I remember her asking, "So those were the things that you found pre-surgery, right?" and the doctor replying "yes." She went on to ask, "So she no longer has cancer?" and my doctor said, "No." With a confused expression look from my sister to me, my doctor soon realized that up until that moment I thought she was telling me that I still had cancer. "She said I'm so sorry I thought you knew that's what I was telling you." She touched my leg and said, "You are cancer free." That's when the breath that I didn't realize I was holding released.

Post Operation with my Plastic Surgeon

I had an appointment with my plastic surgeon who told me that he inserted the expanders during surgery and put my first dosage of cc's inside. He went on to explain that at the next several appointments he would be inserting fluid into the expander so that my breast tissue wouldn't deflate while going through radiation. The scary part is that this would be done by a needle that would be shot into my breast.

Post Operation with my Oncologist

I was nervous when I showed up for this appointment. At my other two appointments, I'd either was told news that I didn't expect or had something done that I didn't expect so I was unsure what would happen. I thought about my friend's appointment and how she was told by her oncologist that she would have to have chemo so I was hoping that I wouldn't have to hear the same thing. Unfortunately, that wasn't the case because I was told that he wanted me to take another round of chemo. I was told that this time around I would be able to receive my chemo orally which meant that I would be able to take a chemo pill from the convenience of my own home. He told me that I would have to take it for 18 weeks. Again, he was talking, and I had tuned out. I was hurt to hear that I was being told that I would have to take chemo again. The sucky thing was that it was possible that with the oral chemo I may suffer some of the same side effects as I did the first time around. I had just started to grow my hair back, and now all I could think about was having to lose it again.

While I wanted to ask the Lord why, I knew it was pointless. Because he doesn't make mistakes I knew what was happening to me was all part of his plan.

Chapter 11 - Expansion Appointments

First Expansion Appointment

This was one of my scariest appointments. Not because of what would happen but because of the pain that I knew that I would experience at this appointment. I was scheduled to get my last two tubes out and to have my first two injections of the 100 ccs of fluids per breast. I made it to my scheduled appointment a few minutes early. My husband and I waited in the waiting room for me to be called. He read one of the magazines that was sitting on the table closest to him while I continued to dread what was to come. The nurse called my name, and we followed her back to one of the examining rooms. I walked in and instantly was afraid when I glanced at the four syringes that were filled with 50 cc's each. I was given a gown to change into from the waist up and was told that the doctor would be in shortly. The doc came in and checked to make sure my wounds were healing properly before leaving his nurse to remove my two remaining tubes and to give me my first injection.

I was petrified thinking about how painful it would be to have the tubes removed. The nurse stood in front of me and told me to watch her as she pulled the tubes out at once instead of one at a time. It all happened so fast that I didn't have time to be afraid. Thank God that it wasn't painful and I thank her for doing it the way she did or else I'd continue to stress for no reason.

She used a small magnet catcher to locate the spot on my breast where she needed to stick the needle of fluid into for me to receive my first injection. The way she explained it the edge of the flap that was inserted in me had a magnet on it, and that's where she needed to stick the needle in to inject the fluid to expand it. Once she located the spot, she marked it on my skin with a sharpie marker. I know my blood pressure was probably skyrocketing high because the entire time she was looking for the spot I was thinking about the pain. My sister told me that when she had this done her breast was numb, so she didn't feel anything. I prayed the same thing should happen to me and my prayers were answered because I hardly felt anything when the nurse inserted the needle in my breast. Because I was still numb, I didn't feel the needle go in either breast.

Before leaving the doctor told me that my breasts would feel full either that night or the next day. I had no idea what he was talking about until it happened. It started off feeling like it does after you have a baby and your breast are full of milk then it went to two full breast of pain. They were stiff and heavy, and I couldn't get any comfort like I did after childbirth where I was able to take a shower to release the fullness. This feeling that I was experiencing wasn't going anywhere until it was ready and there was nothing that I could do to help except take pain meds. I was taking hydrocodone and muscle relaxers as prescribed, and the only thing I got from taking them was an upset stomach and at times drowsiness that I couldn't relieve myself off by taking a nap. I couldn't take a nap because I could never get comfortable enough to fall asleep. This went on until my next injection appointment.

Second Expansion Appointment

I had another 100 ccs of saline injected. I made sure to tell them about all of the pain that I experienced over the previous week. I was given a different prescription, and I was told that things would get better over time. It took a few days but the pain eventually lightened up, but I still suffered from being uncomfortable. No matter where I was or what position I was in, I was unable to get comfortable. I remember going to the movies with my family and being uncomfortable the entire time. I only felt comfortable when I was sitting in the recliner in my room. I would sit in that chair until it was time for bed.

It was at this appointment that I ran into my friend J who was also there to get saline injected into her expander. While we had been doing a lot of texting, we hadn't been able to meet up, so it was so good to see her. We talked about everything that we had been through and what we still had left to go through. We made plans to meet up within the next couple of weeks. Unfortunately, we never got the chance to.

Thank God I made it through that visit and scheduled an appointment for the excitement to start all over again the next week which was my last injection appointment. I was told that we would discuss my reconstruction appointment which would take place at least 30 days after my last radiation appointment. I put another timeline on myself by telling myself that my battle would be finished once I finished my reconstructive surgery. Little did I know, that was far from the truth. Not only would I have to have a couple more reconstructive surgeries but for the rest of my life, I would have to live with the possibility of a reoccurrence.

Chapter 12 - Radiation – March 20, 2018

At my first radiation appointment, I was signed in at the front desk and told to sit and wait in the finance department. I sat down with the finance department to discuss payments for my treatments. Thank God that my out of pocket was met with my insurance company. I was told that I wouldn't be responsible for making any out of pocket payments for my treatments. After everything that I had been through, it was a great feeling to know that I wouldn't have to rack up more bills that I wasn't in a position to pay. Again I was dressed in the ugly hospital gown and laying on top of a bed. I laid under a machine that would be scanned around my body, and the rays would radiate my breast and lymph nodes where the cancer was. The ladies explained how they would be putting dots on my body, and those dots would be used every visit to indicate where to place the machine in place over my body for me to receive the best treatment. Then I was told that the mark would be tattooed onto my body. Again, the girl afraid of needles was being told that she would need to be stuck with another needle. I almost jumped to my feet in worry. "Uhh, no one told me that I would have to get a tattoo. What type of tattoo are we talking?" I asked. I was told that it was just a small mark that would only be noticeable by a trained eye. That didn't really give me the comfort that I needed. My issue was not about having a permanent mark on my body. By now my body was covered with bruises and scars from all of the treatment. My main concern was the pain that I would have to endure to get those marks. After noticing how uncomfortable I was about getting the marks tattooed, I was told that they could use a permanent marker to make the mark instead. "Yes, I was down for anything that didn't require a needle." The only catch with the marker was that I would have to take special care not to get the marks wet because if they were washed off, the entire process would have to be restarted and that could extend my radiation period. That sucked because my family had a Springbreak trip planned to SeaWorld Aquatica that weekend. I knew that they only way I could ensure that the marks didn't wash off was to avoid water; therefore, I wouldn't be able to swim.

For the most part, my radiation appointments went along without a problem. As soon as I was called to the back, I would get dressed in my hospital gown and go for my procedure which normally took 15 minutes, and I was out. I was told by the nurses and the doctors to put on a recommended dosage of lotion on per day, and if I am being honest, I didn't. Some days I didn't put on any, and that was not a good decision on my part.

It was the last week of radiation before I started noticing radiation burns. That's when I talked to J who told me how important the lotion was and to make sure my armpit was aired out after each treatment. I experienced a ton of burning sensations and actual burns under my armpits that could have been avoided if I knew to air them out. I'm sure I would have figured this out myself if I'd conducted my own research over radiation but like with chemo I was too scared to know. I was scared to hear about others experience with radiation because I didn't want my brain to trick me into those being my reactions. Instead of researching, I decided it was best to just pray my way through any obstacle that may come my way. This helped me because I didn't go through my treatment waiting for the things to happen that I read. Instead, I took it one day at a time while praying extra hard when my comfort level changed. I knew that I would experience burns, I just didn't know when and how bad.

I remember my mom experiencing forehead burns a week after having radiation for the legions that had spread to her brain. The pain in her head had become unbearable, so her oncologist suggested giving her radiation in an effort to shrink the tumors.

This did help, but the cancer that spread all over her body overshadowed her relief.

A couple of days after I finished my radiation was when my skin turned for the worse. I had burn marks and blisters that seemed to pop up overnight. I thank God the burns didn't come until I finished my treatment but seeing the dark burns was a total shock and to say the burns were uncomfortable was an understatement. Because I went so long without getting any burns, I thought I had defied the odds and wouldn't get any but I was wrong. The burns turned darker and spread wider by the day, and they also became more painful. The burn started above my right breast and spread to my shoulder. Soon after, I started noticing that my underarm was a scary black color and that there was a painful blister in the center of my underarm: not a musty stench but a weird, different smell. On top of having to worry about the physical and mental aspect of the burns, I dealt with the emotional side of having the burns. After a recommendation from my sister, I used Domeboro for the blisters, and it truly helped.

I thank God that I didn't get the burns until after my treatments ended but there were painful and somewhat unbearable. It was strange to wake up daily and see that the burns had spread wider. While receiving the radiation, I would have to lay on the bed and stretch both of my arms above my head and hold onto a bar that was overhead. I had no complaints in the beginning, but it became painful towards the end.

The pain from the burns went away after a few weeks. The physical scars have yet to leave.

Reality check – April 23, 2018

I was at my son's basketball practice when I received a text from J. Since we texted each other weekly to update each other about our condition, I assumed that's what her text was in regards to. Last time we talked, we discussed her finishing her radiation treatments a couple of days before mine, so I assumed that her text was to give me the heads up on how she felt and what to expect. When I opened her text I was shocked to read her message letting me know that she was scheduled have to have another biopsy performed because of a concerning spot that the doctor saw on her liver. Until I received that text from her, I didn't realize that I had to worry about a reoccurrence so soon after chemo. I was shocked that the doctors that it was possible for her to have cancer and for it to possibly have spread to another part of her body when she completed every step of her treatment plan. A treatment plan to me was a roadmap to being cancer-free. Until to that point, I felt like as long as I did everything that was requested of me to be a survivor then I would be a survivor. J possibly being diagnosed again so soon after her surgery proved that logic wrong. As far as I knew, she was taking the chemo pill and radiation. I began wondering what more I could do to avoid a reoccurrence.

With us going through every step together I was making her possible diagnosis mine which was the wrong move to make because I drove myself crazy. I had to remember my mom always saying what is for me is for me. She would say your name is Tamara and not "whomever" it was that I was comparing myself to. I spent the next few days trying to calm my nerves of what could be. This was when I first realized how much my life would change and that there was nothing that I could do about it. I would no longer have a calming feeling when it came to my health. Every possible issue would send me into panic mode.

Several days after getting that text from her, I received another text that she got the results of her biopsy and the doctor's concern was validated. My friend was diagnosed twice with cancer within a year, and this time she was diagnosed with liver cancer. The wind was knocked out of me after I read her text. I spent most of that day and the next crying. I was once again feeling two emotions. I felt guilty, and sadness with my friend like I previously did while going through my mom's battle with cancer. I felt sad because I knew how hard it had to be for her and her family to receive that news again when she wasn't finished fighting her initial battle. I was scared of losing her, and at the same time, I felt guilty to be thanking God that I wasn't dealing with what she was. I felt it was selfish for me to be happy about my diagnosis while she was diagnosed again. I remember telling my son about J and him saying, "Mom I am so sorry for your friend and her family, and we have to pray for her, but I'm happy it's not you." He asked if he was wrong for feeling like that. What could I tell him when I was having those feelings myself.

Unlike my sister, when I was diagnosed with cancer, I went out of my way to avoid support groups or establish relationships with cancer patients for this exact reason. I didn't ever want to meet and lose a friend. Now regardless of how hard I tried to separate myself, I was in a position that I had a close friend that could possibly be losing her battle. Like I've been told by others, sometimes God brings people in your life for either their sake or yours. I felt like God brought J in my life to benefit me. I learned a lot from her. She kept me strong when I was beginning to weaken. There were times when she was going through it, but her attitude was so positive and her fight was still present. Her strength motivated me.

It hurt because J was another person that I knew I was getting ready to lose while going through this storm. I hadn't known J long, but I knew her long enough to know that like my mother, J was a good person. I also knew that like my mother, J was getting ready to be called home and there was nothing that I could do about it. What I learned about J in the short time that I knew her was that she was a God fearing woman. She was also a fighter who endured every treatment possible to prevent a reoccurrence, and it still happened. Watching her go through this reoccurrence reminded me of myself. I always told everyone that knowing that I did all that I could to fight this battle would give me peace and I could tell that it gave her peace too.

After my initial shock of her being diagnosed, we both talked about keeping the faith. My friend told me that her prognosis was not good and that her oncologist recommended that she try seeking treatment from MD Anderson which is a big cancer treatment center in Houston, Texas. Hearing that she was being diagnosed again when we weren't finished with our current treatment plan was heartbreaking. All I could do was pray for her and her family. It was scary to know that someone going through the same treatment plan as myself was being re-diagnosed and so soon.

In a panic, I called my doctor's office to see if there was anything that I could do that I wasn't already doing. I asked if I should start the oral chemo pill sooner than planned. After calming me, I was told that there was no reason to double my treatment. I was also told that we would discuss my treatment options at my next appointment that was scheduled the following week and to try to take it easy and not stress out until then. I knew that would be impossible. I had to continuously remind myself over the next week that God is and will always be in control. Reminding myself this helped me stay sane but I'd be lying if I said that the flesh didn't continue to make me want to doubt the faith that I was raised to lean on.

While I entertained taking the pill and radiation together, I knew it served no purpose. J was taking them both when she was diagnosed. The radiation may have prevented the cancer from coming back in her breast, but it didn't protect her liver. I knew that I had to lean on God and my faith had to be stronger now than ever so I continued to talk to the Lord and ask him for the strength to make it through the process. I knew that there was no reason to stress over the things that I couldn't control because God wouldn't allow anything to happen that wasn't supposed to happen.

A few weeks after I finished my radiation, I started having hot flashes. My night sweats had gotten really bad. I started back using the fan on my bedside that I used when I was taking the Lupron shot, and it had been 4 months since I had my last shot. Those hot flashes reminded me of the feelings I had right before I was diagnosed. I had problems sleeping through the night and would wake up in the middle of the night tossing and turning because of the hot flashes. With everything that was going on with my friend who was diagnosed, I worried that the hot flashes was a sign that the cancer had returned. I prayed to God that everything was good and that my hot flashes were being caused by all of the poison that was being injected into my system leaving my body.

Thinking about starting the chemo pill was also stressing me. I worried about the effects of it and the possibility of losing my hair again. My hair had just started growing back, and I was loving it. The thought of losing it again made me feel like I was taking a step back instead of the step towards my mission. I often listened to a Motivational Speaker who once said: "You are either getting ready to go into a storm, in a storm, or coming out of a storm." Unfortunately, I was feeling like I would never get to enjoy the coming out stage because I was steadily being pushed into another storm and it had become depressing. I tried my hardest to keep my faith strong and continue to leave what I was going through in God's hands, but it was hard.

Fighting my battle with cancer was so hard because even when I was too tired to move, I had no choice but to move because my family needed me. My kids needed to be picked up from school, taken to dental and doctors' appointments, and basketball practices and games. During those hard times where I wanted to just give up, I knew that I couldn't so I just prayed harder for strength. There were days when I wanted to just jump on the floor like a child and throw a tantrum, but I knew that I couldn't. I knew that I couldn't let my family see me lose control. As long as I was strong, they would be. I thank God that I had my faith because I'm not sure I would have made it without it.

Mom's 66th Birthday - May 6, 2018

Celebrating my mother's first birthday without her here on this earth was so hard. To honor her, my siblings and I came together and had a cookout. Being with family made it more bearable, but I still missed my mother like crazy. For the most part, we laughed and shared memories of her. In her honor, our whole family released balloons for her that day in Texas, Arkansas, Mississippi, and Illinois. It was so sad celebrating her birthday without her, but it was easier to end it laughing with my family then by crying. I missed my mom like crazy, but I knew she wasn't coming back so I could either lay around all day crying or get up and enjoy this day celebrating her, so I chose the second option.

Chapter 13 – Xeloda/Radiation Recall

First Three Month Check

On May 9, 2018, I was finally sitting in my oncologist's office for my first 3-month check. I was so nervous. At this appointment, I would get the results of my blood work and I would make a decision on whether taking another round of chemo was best for me or skipping it and going along to a hormone blocker. After everything that was going on with my friend, I was afraid to get the results of my blood work. From the time I dropped my kids off at school until I left for my doctor's office, I walked the floor making myself a nervous wreck. The fear had set in so bad that I was short of having a nervous breakdown. The fear had me crying on and off. Although I prayed to my God for a 100% healing, the flesh was taking over and I was worried. Even though I felt like I was 100% healed, my brain kept playing the "what if" game with me. I prayed over and over for strength.

Deciding on taking another round of chemo or Tamoxifen was a hard decision for me. All I could think about was the fact that my grandmother refused a second round of chemo and her cancer reoccurred. After several of months of her going in and out of the hospital we lost her. I even thought about the fact that J was taking a second round of chemo when she was diagnosed with cancer in another part of her body. I was at a crossroad where I could either decide to take the chemo pill and have a bigger chance of beating a reoccurrence or I could decide not to take the chemo pill and risk being in a situation like my grandma. I was told that my grandmother had cancer cells that had traveled to other parts of her body that could have been washed away if she'd taken the chemo.

This helped me realize that when it came to making decisions about cancer treatments, there is no right answer there is only a right answer for me. I knew that while going through this journey, I would have to be ok with making decisions that may not have a 100% success rate or decisions that would put my mind at ease. I knew that I'd have to learn to make the decisions that I could live with and not worry about the decisions that were construed to be the "right decisions" because honestly, no one knows the right decisions.

I realized then that I was living a life that even if I did everything that I was instructed to do, the inevitable could happen and I could have a reoccurrence. From that day, I decided that instead of stressing about obstacles that came my way, I would pray to God that they didn't.

I thank God that all of the tests from my bloodwork came back good that day. I didn't receive the results of my tumor marker that appointment because I was told that it takes longer than the other tests, so the results were not back by the time I left the office. My doctor told me that he would call me as soon as he received my results. He told me that he was a little concern about my results because at my last appointment my numbers were higher than they should have been being that I had already had chemo and the surgery. I was shocked to hear him say that because I had no idea it was a concern of his. His concern soon become a concern of my own. I guess it was a good thing that I didn't know about it following my previous surgery because I would have been a wreck the entire time between my two appointments.

My doctor discussed my options when it came to my hormone blocker medication which confused me because I had it in my mind that we would discuss the chemo and if we decided that it wasn't the right route for me to take then we would discuss the hormone blocker. He was skipping a step, and I let him know. He said he was hesitant to bring up the chemo because he thought I had ruled that option out last time we talked. He also said that he was concerned for me to start the chemo pill because the effects were hard for some of his patients. He said he had patients who took the medication and struggled the entire time and they were emotionally and physically sound before starting the treatment. Because of what I'd been through emotionally and physically over the last year he was afraid that mentally I wouldn't be able to handle it. Hearing him say that I may be too weak to take the pill made me feel challenged and everyone who knows me know that I can't forego a challenge.

He said my reaction to him bringing up the chemo pill when we last met had him thinking I was emotionally spent. In my defense, hearing that I had to take more chemo "was a shock." Back in February when I met with my oncologist post operation, I came in with my spirits high. I was a woman who had just endured months of chemo, I had lost my mother to cancer a couple of months prior, and I had just had a double mastectomy. I was tired. I thought that all I had left to do was endure weeks of radiation and have my reconstructive surgery and I'd be done. At that appointment, I thought I would get my blood results and hear my options when it came to blocking my hormones. After explaining the results of all of my blood work, he went on to discuss my pathology report. He explained that after enduring months of chemo I still had a tumor in my breast and cancer in 1 of 6 lymph nodes that were pulled. He was happy that my tumor had shrunk so drastically, but he was concerned that after taking the 8 rounds of chemo that the cancer was still in my body at the time of the surgery. Knowing that it was removed at surgery gave him little comfort. His way of thinking was that there was a chance that a cancer cell could have broken away and swum to other parts of my body at some point and over time that cancer would grow if it wasn't washed away with the chemo. He said the chemo would give me a higher chance of avoiding a reoccurrence. While he explained percentage rates, I didn't hear any of it because I had tuned him out. My whole body was numb. All I could think was "As hard as I fought the previous year, it wasn't enough." Through teary eyes, I thanked my doctor for all of the information even though I didn't actually hear it before telling him that I didn't think another round of chemo was where I wanted to go. I told him that my husband and I would pray to God and have an answer for him when we met again. I guess he took my reaction as a defeat when in all reality it was an "I wasn't ready to hear what he told me" reaction.

When I sat in his office for the second time that year, I had finished radiation, and I had more energy than I did the first time and my fighter instinct was back. I knew that I wanted to do everything that I needed to do to prevent a reoccurrence and that included taking this preventive chemo. Like I previously stated, I wanted to always look into my children's eyes and say I gave it my all. I didn't feel like I could do that if I didn't at least give the chemo a try. I knew I could always stop it and walk away if any complications arose, so I told my doc that I wanted to give it a try.

My mom's favorite saying was for me to find someone who I had favor with when. This meant that I needed to find the person that was Godsent to me to make it through an obstacle. I definitely felt like my oncology doctor was Godsent and I knew in order for me to make it through this journey, I had to remember he was Godsent and follow his lead. I asked him to give me the recommendation about chemo that he would give his wife, and he told me that he'd tell his wife to give it a try and that she could always quit if she had any complications. After asking my husband what he thought and getting his response, "whatever you decide I got your back. If you want to do it, then let's do it" I decided I would do it. We discussed the pill and the benefits of taking it. My doctor knew that I wasn't a 100% with taking the chemo so he said that we should fast and pray until the following week and I'd start the pill unless God said otherwise. We finished that appointment in prayer like we had all of the previous ones. This journey is hard enough, so I am so happy that I was being led by a doctor that I felt was Godsent. Doing so definitely took some of the pressure off of me.

Following that appointment, I worried about my tumor results until I received a call from my doctor. He called me back that night to give me the results of my test. I'm guessing he was multi-tasking because he said my name and waited a few minutes after I responded to continue talking. Those seconds felt like hours. That was time enough for me to run a million thoughts through my head. "What if he had bad news to share and he was taking a moment to word it right" was the biggest thought I had running through my head. I almost screamed at him to "please get it out." I made up my mind then that I would ask him to work his visits backwards. He was so thorough that I was about to pass out by the time he got to the important part of the appointment, and the suspense killed me. It was the whole meat and potato concept. He was busy giving me the potato part of my condition when I was more interested in the meat of it which is if the cancer had returned. I mostly wanted to hear if things changed more than anything else so I'd rather he tell me about the cancer before discussing other things like iron levels.

When he finally spoke, he started by saying "I have some good news for you" and those were the best words that I'd heard in a while. I didn't know exactly what he had to tell me but a doctor calling me with good news was foreign after the year that I had. He told me that my tumor marker numbers were back normal meaning that there was no sign that I had a tumor in my body. It felt good to be able to share the good news with my family for once.

Knowing that I'd never have that peace of knowing that I once had at the doctor's appointments, I thanked God for this one.

Goodbye J

I was on the way to my son's end of the year celebration at school with my children in the car when I looked down at my phone and saw J's name on my caller ID. J and I normally communicated by text and not phone calls, so I was shocked that she was calling and not texting but I never expected to hear what I did. When I last spoke to her she told me that the chemo wasn't working because the cancer had spread to another organ. She also said that she was having breathing issues which reminded me of my mother towards the end of her battle.

Knowing about all of this, I knew when I saw her name on the screen that it was not good news, but I was not prepared for the news that I got.

I answered my phone and prepared to speak to my friend but instead I heard her husband's voice. He called to let me know that my partner in this battle was no longer fighting. He informed me that she had passed away during the night. I wasn't ready to hear what he had to say and my world stopped for at least 30 seconds. I struggled to comprehend what he was telling me. I'm sure he knew how much what he told me affected me by my response. There was no way that another fighter with what my mom called "pit-bull faith" was called home. After being able to get out the words to offer him my condolence, I broke down in tears on the phone before hanging up. I was full of so many emotions. Like with the loss of my mother, I knew I had to be strong. I was finally at my son's school, and the last thing that he needed was to worry about his mother. Seeing me hang up the phone in tears had already affected him, and it was evident that his mood had changed. After parking and telling my husband about the loss of my friend, I dried my tears before going in and acting as if I had not just been given bad news. I knew that crying would only make me weak and unable to continue my battle. I had to start my new prescription of the chemo pill the following week and I needed to be strong because I had no idea how my body would react from it.

Like my mother, J died within a year after she was diagnosed. Like my mother, J had that mustard seed faith. I remember talking to her about the struggles that were making me weak and her saying that we needed to pray for strength and we did. I remember how upbeat she was when she told me about her reoccurrence. Even though she received news that would make the strongest person weak she still sounded strong. I was sad and angry, and she was talking with words full of faith. Seeing her full of so much faith and strength was helpful to me because it made me fight harder on my weak days. If she could do it, then I knew I could too.

To be at my strongest, I knew that I needed to talk to God about my issue with doing all that I could do to stay cancer free. I wanted to do everything imaginable but after seeing what happened to my friend I had to accept that I could do it all and still be diagnosed again. I knew that I had to accept and live with the belief that God is always going to allow what he is going to allow and that there is nothing that I can do about it. Because of that, I've decided to enjoy life and live every day like it could be my last.

Began my treatment of the Xeloda (chemo) pill

I began my dosage of Xeloda in May of 2018. I was told that I needed to take 5 pills at a time once a day. The first 5 rounds went smooth. I didn't have any issues. The sixth week is when I noticed a rash that started spreading up and down my breast bone. I had the rash on my shoulder and over onto my back. I began conducting my research and scaring myself thinking about a possible cancer reoccurrence. I read somewhere that a rash could mean that there was a possible reoccurrence. I called my oncologist and spoke with someone who was not my doctor's nurse because she happened to be out that day. I was told that it was possibly a heat rash. I was familiar with a heat rash, so I knew that it was not that, but because she wasn't giving me the dreaded news I got a year ago, I was happy to let her give me a wrong diagnosis. After several of days trying different rash creams, I decided to call my radiation doctor because I realized that the rash wasn't getting any better and that it happened to be in the same spot that I received radiation. I was told by the nurse that my rash and the discoloration of my breast was concerning. I had finished radiation a couple of months back so she told me that the rash should be better and not worse. Until she said that, I hadn't realized that my breast not healing was an issue because I heard that it took a while. I just assumed that it was going through the stages like my doctor told me that it would.

Radiation Recall

Later that day, my doctor called and told me that what I was experiencing was called "Radiation Recall." He explained that radiation recall happened to some patients who took Xeloda after having radiation. He explained that radiation recall meant that the effects of radiation was being recalled. "Thank you Jesus!" I was comfortable with that explanation. He prescribed me a topical steroid cream to heal the rash. The cream helped the rash go away within a couple of weeks but the discoloration never did. My oncologist thought it was best for me to stop the chemo until the rash completely cleared. I was told that it might take months to heal so we discussed me stopping the Xeloda and going straight to the hormone blocker - Tamoxifen. I was ok with this because before deciding to take the Xeloda I said I would try it and if I had any problems then I would take it as a sign from God that it wasn't for me. I prayed to God to lead me to the right decision.

Like I've told anyone dealing with cancer or a caretaker for someone dealing with cancer, you have to do what you are comfortable with because no one knows the right thing to do. We only know what may help. If you decide not to take chemo and you are comfortable with that decision, then please don't. I was comfortable doing everything within reason to beat this battle.

I thank God that I was able to take trips while taking this medication but because of it my experiences were different from the trips that we took the year before.

Trip to Vegas

My husband and I took a trip to Vegas a couple of months before I was diagnosed. We enjoyed it and said that we would repeat it the following summer. Needless to stay, our trip to Las Vegas the second time around was nowhere near as fun as the first time. Because of the medication that I was taking, I had been instructed to stay out of the sun. The weather was 100+ the entire time that we were there. This meant that we stayed indoors at different casinos most of the day. When we were outdoors, I tired quickly. I was told that I could have a drink or two while on the medication, but I decided that I wouldn't. All of this was a difference from the first time around. I thank God for blessing me with the opportunity to revisit Vegas but I was beginning to accept the fact that my body was not aligned with my brain. My brain told me that I was ok but my body told me something completely different.

Family Cruise to Mexico

Every year we try to take the kids on a trip. Because of all of the treatment that I had endured, we decided that we would do something with the kids that wouldn't be strenuous or out in the sun so we decided on a cruise. We'd been hearing about how exciting taking a cruise was so we decided to do that. I knew that I would have to take things a little easy because of how things went in Vegas so I decided that I would stay indoors most of the time. The pool was on the deck so I knew I could sit in the shade when I sat out with the kids but that I would have to avoid the sun. Around 30 minutes after being in our room on the cruise ship we were told that there would be a safety meeting that wouldn't take long. We all had designated places we had to stand and hear the safety presentation. Unfortunately, our cruise was leaving from New Orleans in August so to say it was hot was an understatement. After 15 minutes of standing in a line in a hot room with people standing in front and back of me for the safety meeting, I started to feel dizzy. While praying to God that this meeting would hurry and end, I began swaying as I felt myself falling to the ground. All I remember is the panic in the voices of my husband, daughter, and son while I laid there. No matter how hard I tried to fake being ok I couldn't. My body was too weak to be in control. My husband began fanning me while other guests crowded around asking if I was ok. I was finally able to open my eyes after a few minutes of fanning. I saw fear when I looked into the faces of my kids. Even though I didn't have the strength, I knew I had to get up. After a few minutes, someone came over with a glass of cold water which helped. After a few more minutes, I was able to stand up and walk out of that area into an air-conditioned room. Again, this trip was not like the trip that we took last year before I was diagnosed. Everything was changing and I had to be ok with that. Pushing myself was only making things worse. I knew that I had to give my body time it needed to heal so I took it easy for the rest of that cruise.

That day I was reminded that my body healed slower than I thought so even though I looked and felt a lot better, I still had a while to go. Thank God that my condition didn't ruin our trip.

Tamara B. Newborn

Personal Reflection: Right before our family trip to California in 2017, I decided that I would seek treatment for my lump. Our family trips are so important to us, so I decided to wait until we came back from California to go. I didn't want to ruin it by receiving bad news. I eventually went to the doctor, received the bad news, and was able to continue living life. When life happens, we have to deal with it and keep it moving.

Chapter 14 - Reconstructive Surgery

Thanksgiving 2018

Thanksgiving was by far one of the hardest days of my life. It was the first Thanksgiving that I had to endure without my mother. I moved away from home years ago, but my mother and I always made an effort to keep in touch as if I was local. It was a tradition for me to call her 50 million times while cooking my holiday meals. Annually, I would ask her the two types of greens that I used, and annually she would have to tell me. This year, it was a reality check when I reached for my phone to ask the types of greens while making my grocery list before remembering she was gone. It was then that I had to accept that trivial things such as calling my mother to ask her about food selections would no longer be a luxury that I would have.

Thank God for family because my sisters and I stood in for my mother for each other. Because we were no longer able to call and ask my mother questions about our Thanksgiving meals, we called each other. My immediate family and I spent the holiday in Mississippi with my sister and her family. All I could think about was the fact that the year before I spent the holiday home while my mother was in the hospital holding on to life. The entire time, we were praying and hoping that my mother would make a miraculous recovery. This year, I was hoping to forget those memories and that sadness. The day was hard but spending it with family helped.

A Year Later

This day was a year since my mother was declared brain dead. For me, it felt like yesterday because I have been stuck in that same spot. Trying to recover from my loss. Following the loss of my mother, I completed my chemo, I had my surgery, and radiation but those things were done purely off of adrenaline. I had yet to feel whole again and doubt that I ever would again. A year after her death and I was still asking myself how I could exist in a world without my mother. I don't question the Lord so I know that if He took her, then it was his purpose. I do question this cruel world that we live in where you are raised in love and then once you are old enough to understand the wholeness of that love, it is snatched away and then you spend the rest of your life trying to heal from that loss and along the way you will lose others that you need to heal from.

Even though I spent the day living like it was any other day it wasn't. It was a year from the worse day of my life. No matter how hard it was for me to live in the present, I couldn't. Most days I wake up and crave a conversation with my mother. On other days, I do whatever I have to do not to think about her. Counseling to deal with my mother's passing would have to wait. I had surgery in a few days, so I knew I had to wait. I didn't want to open up the flood gates and be unable to close them before my surgery. I wanted to be physically, mentally, and emotionally stable when the day came.

I've known people who celebrate two wedding dates. They celebrate the day they get married (usually at the courthouse) and they celebrate the date of their actual wedding. My mother's day of death would be the same. We will remember her on the day that the doctor told us that she was brain dead and we will remember her on the day that she was disconnected from the machine and pronounced dead.

Annually, I could mourn her on those two days or learn to celebrate her by thinking about the good times I shared with her over the years. My mother cared dearly for her family, so I know she wouldn't want me to be sad. In her last days, she went out of her way to pretend to be stronger than what she was for us.

Reconstructive Surgery - December 6, 2018

When the day arrived for my reconstructive surgery, I was so ready to get it over with. I wasn't nervous. I had already prayed to God over the hands and minds of the doctors who would be performing my surgery. I had also prayed that my heart and body would be strong enough to make it through this surgery, so I was ready to go. My husband and I went to the hospital alone, but by the time that I changed into my hospital gown and had an IV put in, my sister, my niece, and my children had arrived.

My family was as happy as I was that the time had arrived. I'm sure they were tired of hearing me complain about being uncomfortable and in pain from the expanders. My surgery being rescheduled two months prior didn't help. Two Months Prior my surgery was canceled, and I was told that it would need to be rescheduled due to complications with my insurance. I had just switched insurance, and they were afraid that it would not be effective on the date of my surgery even though I was told that it would backdate and cover the surgery when it was effective. I spent two days before my scheduled surgery calling around and stressing over the possibility of my surgery being canceled. It was cancelled the night before the morning that my insurance actually went into effect. That had to be one of the most stressful moments during this battle.

After all of the waiting to get this surgery over with, I was so happy that the time had come. My doctor came in before the surgery to make his surgical marks. Once the anesthesiologist came in and gave me my meds, I told my family goodbye while being rolled back for surgery. That was the last thing that I remember.

What felt like 20 minutes later but was actually 7-8 hours, I was looking into the faces of two of my sisters. I remember feeling irritated because I was tired and just wanted to sleep, but the nurses wouldn't let me. They kept shoving a breathing mask in my face. What was a scary moment for one of my sisters wasn't for me. My sister realized that my breathing was off and my heartbeat was beating fast but I didn't nor did I care at the moment. I remember asking for my husband and children because I was slowly going back to sleep and I wanted to see them before I did.

I could hear my nurses and sisters having a conversation back and forth about my heart rate. The nurses were telling them that I was having the same heart issue that I had back in December when I was checked into the hospital. They told them that they would be giving me the same meds that they gave me back in December to slow my heartbeat down and watch me. They also said my blood pressure was up.

I was in a medicated sleep the rest of the night and part of the next day. They gave me the morphine push that I was able to use every 10 minutes to keep the pain away. I used it as needed, and this caused the drowsiness. I remember everything looking blurry and feeling dizzy the first couple of days.

The day after my surgery I was allowed to have the breathing mask removed. The medication had begun working so my heart and breathing issues were better. I wasn't able to get up and do my walk with physical therapy until a couple of days after my surgery. My kids and husband came daily, and my sister stayed the nights.

I had issues standing in the hospital, but I didn't realize how hard it would be for me to care for myself when I got home. It was a couple of weeks before I was able to stand straight. Because I had the stomach surgery everything was pulled tight. The first couple of days were spent with me going from the bed to the bathroom only. Not only was it uncomfortable for me to stand up. I also had to walk super straight. Regardless of the pain and inconvenience following my surgery, I thank God that I made it through.

Today my Daddy was Diagnosed with Prostate Cancer!

When it rains it pours!!! I spent the day that I found out about my father's diagnosis crying like a baby. I should have been healing and happy that my surgery had finally happened and that I was a few days from getting the last few tubes removed from my body. I was sitting on the couch watching tv and trying to get relaxed when I received a text message from my father. I had to double check my screen several times to make sure I was actually reading what I thought I was reading. No matter how hard I tried to deny it, the words were as clear as day. He was texting to let me know that he had been diagnosed with prostate cancer. Several seconds went by before I was able to release the breath that I didn't realize that I was holding.

Before receiving his text, I had finally got to the point where I could exhale and say the storm was ending. I had finished all of my treatment and major surgeries. It was hard living daily without my mother, but I was starting to get used to the idea that she was no longer around. All I could think was that now my father was being told that the battle that my two sisters, my mother, and I fought was now one that he was facing. When the pressure from knowing that became too much, all I could do was cry. After all that I had been through, I was tired. No matter how hard I tried to be strong, I was constantly being knocked down. My mother taught me to never complain about being tired. She felt that saying so would make my body tired, but I couldn't help it. I was weak, tired, scared, hurt, and worried. It took a while, but I remembered that the same God that saved my sisters and I was the same God that would save my father, so I prayed and prayed and prayed.

I DID!

Psalm 118:17 (KJV) – I shall not die, but live, and declare the works of the Lord.

Chapter 15 – I Made it Through the Storm

Being diagnosed with breast cancer has made me a different person. The losses that I endured along the way, have been life changing and having to cope with those losses while going through my battle with cancer was extremely hard, but that made me a stronger person.

I was diagnosed with breast cancer at one of the worse times ever. While there is no good time to be diagnosed with this disease, I was diagnosed several months after my mom was diagnosed with metastatic stage 4 breast cancer. At the time that I was diagnosed, she was taking radiation for cancerous tumors that had spread to her brain. She was in a weakened state, and if I'm being honest, it was the moment that I realized that she was slipping away. Among other things, her energy level had changed drastically. She was hospitalized a few weeks after I was diagnosed because of her low energy level and lack of appetite. During her last days, I sat back and watched as a machine kept her alive. It all came down to either honoring her wishes by keeping her on the machine until God called her home or giving the doctors the ok to take her off the machine.

I was dealing with this at the same time that I was having to wrap my mind around being diagnosed myself. A month later, I sat at my mother's bedside typing while she was losing her battle. I would be lying if I said that it wasn't hard for me to sit there knowing that her fate could possibly one day be my fate, but I knew that my path was already written, so I refused to let fear control my steps and continued to spend her last days with her. I lost my mother while trying to be strong enough to make it through the storm. While fighting this battle, there were times when I needed her nurturing touch and kind words, but I couldn't have any of it because she was fighting a battle of her own.

Knowing that there is a purpose in every painful situation, I tried not to harp too much on my storms, but some days it was hard. I had to make decisions that no one could ever fathom having to make. On days when I was near a breakdown, I prayed to God for the strength to make it through. I learned the power of prayer while going through this storm and there were plenty of days where I had to let go and let God.

Chapter 16 – Things I learned while Going through the Storm

While going through the storm won't be easy, I hope these little nuggets of advice will make it easier for you while going through it. Below are things that I learned along the way:

1. **Blessing in your Pain.**

   While going through the storm always remember that there is a purpose in your pain. Yes, there will be plenty of hard days so on those days just remember that you are going through this storm for a reason. I set out to find out why I was diagnosed and at such a young age. While I'll never know God's reasons, I find comfort in these two things:

   a. Being diagnosed gave my family a distraction while the matriarch of our family was being called home. It hurt so bad to lose her, and I'm unsure if the pain will ever go away, but I know for a fact that losing her would have been so much harder if I wasn't going through a battle of my own.

   b. I have a story that can help others. I will not live like a victim but a victor. I want people to know that yes the fight is hard but that they can make it through too.

2. **Don't just go through it, Grow through It.**

   In life, we will go through a ton of storms. I feel like there is always something that we can learn about ourselves while going through it. When I was first diagnosed, I wondered why God was allowing me to go through this storm, but through it, I was put in a situation where I had to lean solely on Him. Through this storm, I was also able to teach my children to do the same. While I will always have their backs, I want them to always remember that it is He above who they should lean on when times get hard. I thank my mother for that lesson because I don't know how else I would have made it through this storm.

3. Lean on the Man Above.

Another thing that I've learned while going through the storm is not to put too much faith in man because it is He who has the final say. There were times while going through the storm when I wanted my medical staff to tell me that everything would be ok and that once I finished this fight against cancer that I would be forever healed but they couldn't, and because they couldn't, there were days that I felt empty. I wondered if I was making the right move by enduring months of chemo, losing my hair, gaining weight, feeling weak, and just someone other than myself when there was no certainty that I wouldn't have to endure the same thing again. Thank God for reminding me that He has the final say and because I knew that he was in control, I refused to live in fear. A survivor once said she is living as if she will be forever healed and if she ever found out that she was diagnosed again she will just fight again. Thinking like her put my mind at ease.

4. Your Breast will never be the same.

My sister and I had a conversation last night about life after breast cancer, and we talked about the scars that have been left behind after our breast cancer diagnosis. We both opted to have the DIEP Flap surgery. With this procedure, the surgeon transfers fat from one part of our body to our breast. I am halfway through my process, and she has been done for at least 5 years, but we both agree that the end results is not what we were thinking. When I was first diagnosed, I had a lot of people tell me that coming out of this storm I would have the perk of having better breast but so far that has not been the case. What I have is a tarnished version of what I expected but instead of dwelling on this, I chose to dwell on the fact that I am blessed to be living.

5. There is no 100% guarantee.

In order to make it through this storm emotionatlly sane, I had to accept that there is nothing that I can do to give myself a 100% guarantee that I won't be diagnosed with cancer again. It sucks, and it's a scary thing but it is my new reality. Instead of stressing over things I have no control over, I've decided to pray!

6. Their situation is not your situation.

Now that you are diagnosed it will seem like every time you turn around somebody else is either diagnosed or passes away from cancer but always remember that their situation is not your situation. While going through this storm, I had to make sure that I didn't let other people's end results become my own. I lost my mother, my friend, and attended a funeral for my husband's grandmother while going through treatment. All three ladies were affected by cancer so to see them go was both sad and scary for me. I had to keep telling myself that just because it happened to them did not mean that it was going to happen to me.

7. You are good.

There will be a number of days that you will have to tell yourself that even though you don't feel good, you will. There will be days that you have to remind yourself that "in spite of what you look like that you are good." There were plenty of days where I was super tired, and I gained weight while taking chemo treatments thanks to the steroids that I took. I made it through those hard days by telling myself that I would one day be good again and you have to remind yourself of the same. Always remember that how you feel today has nothing on how you will feel tomorrow. It will get better.

8. Go with the Flow.

A major mistake that I made was thinking that I had control of the situation. I thought that putting time limits on how long this storm would last would make it easier. First, I told myself that I would be finished with all treatments by the one year mark and boy was I wrong. To accomplish this goal, I told myself that I would be finished with chemo within three months. Not only did I not finish in three months but I had to endure a second round of chemo. I told myself that I would have my double mastectomy, radiation, and reconstructive surgery completed within a 6 month period and again I was wrong. I ended up having my reconstructive surgery one month shy of the year mark of my mastectomy surgery. All of these things that didn't line up with the times that I had set only caused me unnecessary stress. I wish I would have realized then what I realize now which is I was never in control. God allowed things to happen in his time. I've definitely learned the true meaning of "God speed."

9. Family Involvement.

Following my second chemo treatment, I started losing my hair, so I decided it was best for me to shave what was left. I left at it as being the best idea but I failed to look at how big of a deal this transformation would be on my children when I went into the bathroom with hair and came out bald. I wish I would have had a discussion with them before cutting my hair bald and my reason for doing so. I did it to stay strong but I failed to realize that even this wasn't their storm directly, they were also going through this storm. From that point on, I involved my family as much as I could. If I could do it over again, I'd let my family be a part of the process of cutting my hair because that was our first major change.

10. Effect on my Family.

A cancer diagnosis may only be given to one person but the effects of that diagnosis is one that the entire family suffers. The decisions that you make will affect them. Yes, they will witness a lot of hard days that you will have to endure but they will also witness God's miracle when you beat this disease.

11. Fear of a Reoccurrence.

Yes, sometimes I fear a reoccurrence but for the most part, I've decided to accept that all of the treatment that I endured to become a survivor was enough to heal me from cancer forever. For the most part, I try not to think about it as nothing more than an illness. Not thinking about the severity of the condition helps me. I know it won't be an easy thing to deal with if it comes back, but I know it's something that I am capable of doing. I choose not to think of the different areas that it may come back in if it returns because it serves no purpose. If the good Lord decides it is my time to go, then there is nothing that I can do about it; therefore, I refuse to spend my days stressing over the "what-ifs."

This whole ordeal has made me a stronger person. My sister and I fought cancer while losing our mother. If I made it through those days, I feel like I can make it through anything. I know whatever storm comes my way, I have what it takes to weather it. No, it won't be easy, but I know for a fact that it can be done. I was spared which means I need to be enjoying myself and living my best life!

12. Medical Dream Team

Going through this storm is hard enough, so I recommend that anyone who is going through it have the best medical staff on their team. Knowing that my medical staff was God sent, I was able to follow my doctors' lead when it came to the hard decisions.

13. Make your Next Step your Best Step.

While fighting this battle, you will have to make choices that not everyone will understand but please do what is best for you because it is you who will have to suffer the consequences. Before I was a patient, I thought I knew what was best for a cancer patient. Now, after being diagnosed I now know that there are no guarantees so I recommend anyone going through this storm to do what makes life easiest and leave the rest in God's hands.

14. When God Speaks, Listen.

I've met people while going through this storm that told me that God talked to them and told them not to take chemo. I recommend that if that's what he said, listen. My mother repeated the exact saying over and over, and because I couldn't understand God's power initially, I asked her to get chemo against his will. She was asked to take chemo treatments by family, friends, and medical staff and for months she stood her ground and said no to chemo. I think the pressure may have become too much for her because she eventually decided that she would take chemo, and it seems like a week after deciding she'd take it, she was hospitalized and soon after slipped into a coma. She eventually took her last breath a couple of months later. I believe that my mother left this world when it was time for her to leave, but I wonder if her last months would have been spent in a coma if she wouldn't have decided to take chemo.

Chapter 17 - Going Through The Storm

1. Taste buds.

Because I had family members who were diagnosed and endured chemo, I'd heard about their taste buds changing, but I still wasn't ready for the change when it happened to me. The change was so drastic, and I had to forego things that I had come to love. For example, I couldn't drink any pop because of the nasty after taste. As a girl growing up in the Midwest, pop (soda) was always my favorite thing to drink. After my first chemo treatment, I had to learn to do without it.

Before being diagnosed, Mexican food was my favorite but going through chemo I had to limit my intake because it was too spicy. I think the spices in all foods were elevated because of the chemo. The salsa that I had always binged on I no longer enjoyed. The meats were salty.

2. Oral Issues

On top of having taste bud issues, I had a bad oral reaction to the chemo. A couple of days after each chemo treatment my throat would become raw and painful and I would develop mouth sores that also made it a struggle to eat. I was given a mouth wash to gargle but I was only able to keep that up for the first two days before the laziness kicked in. I noticed that the rash only stayed around 2-3 days so I convinced myself that I could handle those 2-3 days without doing the wash. I didn't want to do anything more than I had to while going through treatment. My energy was depleted.

3. Lack of Appetite

On top of my tastebud issues, sore throat and mouth sores, I often had a lack of appetite. When it came to eating, I had no favorites it was all about what I could get down. I was lucky enough not to have nausea issues nor did I ever vomit, but from the stories that I heard from family and friends, I knew that going through chemo, I had to make sure that my body stayed replenished with food and water.

The steroids that I was prescribed gave me the urge to eat even when I didn't want to. It was stressful because I had an urge to eat, but I didn't want to. There were days that I was eating because the urge was there from the steroids, but I wasn't enjoying any of my food. I was literally binging. Throwing back food constantly but none of it was enjoyable. Going through this stage reminded me of my mom and how she would always say that she hated eating but since she knew she had to do so in order to live, she did. I always thought that was the craziest thing because, "who didn't like to eat." Going through chemo, I understood. Sometimes eating was painful, sometimes the food was nasty, and sometimes I just didn't want to eat, but I continued to eat because I knew I had to in order to survive.

4. Hair loss.

I cut my hair prior to starting chemo so I didn't have to endure losing long strands. Instead, I endured pulling back small clumps. Not only did the chemo cause my hair to fall out, it caused the grade of my hair to change. Where my hair was originally soft, the hair that was falling out in clumps was more of a hard and spikey feeling. Everything made my hair fall out. When I ran my fingers through my hair, it would fall out. That was a shock, and it's something that I still suffer from. Now every time that I run my hands through my hair, for a second I fear pulling a handful of hair.

5. Having my Blood Drawn.

I was never comfortable with needles, so my first couple of chemo appointments were rough. By the time I arrived at my appointment I had worried about being stuck so much that I'd almost made myself sick. Thankfully, those first couple of visits I didn't have any issues with having my blood drawn. If anything, I was the problem. I was so scared that I am sure it made it harder on the person trying to take my blood. Towards the end of my chemo treatments, I felt like my veins had either dried up or was just done pumping because it was so hard for the phlebotomists to take my blood. It got so bad that I was told that I should get approval from my doctor to start taking blood from my port. Thankfully, things never got that far.

6. What I dreaded the most about my Chemo Appointments.

While having my blood drawn was always a dreadful thing, it wasn't the most dreaded part of my chemo appointments. The most dreaded part of my chemo appointment was having my port connected to the IV. Three days before I had my first chemo appointment, I had a small port installed inside the skin of my left breast. I was told the port was installed for convenience. Instead of having to hook my IV up to a vein each appointment, they would hook it up to the port. I was given a tube of Lidocaine cream that I was told to apply over the area where my port was installed within an hour before my appointment. The cream was used to numb my skin so that I wouldn't feel the needle of the IV being pushed inside my skin. I was also told to cover the cream with saran wrap to make sure it didn't rub into my clothes and become messy. On the first appointment, I applied the cream as instructed but unfortunately, I felt everything. From that moment on, I dreaded every appointment because I was scared that I would have to endure that type of pain again.

7. Most Memorable Chemo Appointment.

While my first chemo appointment was one that I'll never forget, that wasn't my most memorable appointment. Yes, it was the appointment where I had to accept that I had cancer and that for the next several of months I would have to receive these treatments and because of it my body and appearance would be going through several different changes. My most memorable appointment was my sixth chemo appointment. This was the second appointment where I was given my new chemo medication. I remember being an hour into my treatment when I began feeling spasms in my back. It felt like the pain intensified by the second. At that appointment, I experienced the pain and bad reaction that I always feared.

8. Mindset.

Thank God for giving me the peace of mind to know that while this storm wouldn't be easy, I could make it through. Instead of being scared of what would happen if my chemo didn't work, I concentrated on doing what I had to do to make it through each moment. Instead of looking at what I was going through as the big life ailing illness that it was, I decided to look at it as nothing more than an illness, and with the right medicine, I would be healed.

I thank God that he didn't let those negative thoughts derail my mission. The way I dealt with my journey was with the mindset that as long as I continuously prayed, did what the doctors told me to do, took my chemo, and took care of my body, I would accomplish my goal of beating cancer. Knowing that I was doing all of those things I knew that it was only right that at the end I'd be cancer free. This helped me to keep a clear mind and having a clear mind while going through my battle absolutely helped.

Another thing that my mother used to always say that I never understood until going through this battle is, "I can't let the negative in because I am trying to get a prayer through." While going through this storm, I learned that anything that can derail me from my mission could be negative. If I would have allowed the "what-ifs" into my mind those negative thoughts could have been enough to weaken me and derail me from my mission.

Being in sync with my husband while going through the treatments made it so much easier. We decided in the beginning that we would do everything that we had to do in order to beat this illness and that's what we set out to do. Thank God that we both had the same level of faith because we did a lot of talking to HIM during those days.

Tamara B. Newborn

MAKING IT THROUGH THE STORM

Made in the USA
Columbia, SC
17 June 2019